Achieving Procreation

Fertility, Reproduction and Sexuality

GENERAL EDITORS:

Soraya Tremayne, Founding Director, Fertility and Reproduction Studies Group and Research Associate, Institute of Social and Cultural Anthropology, University of Oxford.

Marcia C. Inhorn, William K. Lanman, Jr. Professor of Anthropology and International Affairs, Yale University.

David Parkin, Fellow of All Souls College, University of Oxford.

Philip Kreager, Director, Fertility and Reproduction Studies Group, and Research Associate, Institute of Social and Cultural Anthropology and Institute of Human Sciences, University of Oxford

Volume 1
Managing Reproductive Life: Cross-Cultural Themes in Fertility and Sexuality
Edited by Soraya Tremayne

Volume 2
Modern Babylon? Prostituting Children in Thailand
Heather Montgomery

Volume 3
Reproductive Agency, Medicine and the State: Cultural Transformations in Childbearing
Edited by Maya Unnithan-Kumar

Volume 4
A New Look at Thai AIDS: Perspectives from the Margin
Graham Fordham

Volume 5
Breast Feeding and Sexuality: Behaviour, Beliefs and Taboos among the Gogo Mothers in Tanzania
Mara Mabilia

Volume 6
Ageing without Children: European and Asian Perspectives on Elderly Access to Support Networks
Edited by Philip Kreager and Elisabeth Schröder-Butterfill

Volume 7
Nameless Relations: Anonymity, Melanesia and Reproductive Gift Exchange between British Ova Donors and Recipients
Monica Konrad

Volume 8
Population, Reproduction and Fertility in Melanesia
Edited by Stanley J. Ulijaszek

Volume 9
Conceiving Kinship: Assisted Conception, Procreation and Family in Southern Europe
Monica M. E. Bonaccorso

Volume 10
Where There is No Midwife: Birth and Loss in Rural India
Sarah Pinto

Volume 11
Reproductive Disruptions: Gender, Technology, and Biopolitics in the New Millennium
Edited by Marcia C. Inhorn

Volume 12
Reconceiving the Second Sex: Men, Masculinity, and Reproduction
Edited by Marcia C. Inhorn, Tine Tjørnhøj-Thomsen, Helene Goldberg, and Maruska la Cour Mosegaard

Volume 13
Transgressive Sex: Subversion and Control in Erotic Encounters
Edited by Hastings Donnan and Fiona Macgowan

Volume 14
European Kinship in the Age of Biotechnology
Edited by Jeanette Edwards and Carles Salazar

Volume 15
Kinship and Beyond: The Genealogical Model Reconsidered
Edited by Sandra Bamford and James Leach

Volume 16
Islam and New Kinship Reproductive Technology and the Shariah in Lebanon
Morgan Clarke

Volume 17
Childbirth, Midwifery and Concepts of Time
Edited by Christine McCourt

Volume 18
Assisting Reproduction, Testing Genes Global Encounters with the New Biotechnologies
Edited by Daphna Birenbaum-Carmeli and Marcia C. Inhorn

Volume 19
Kin, Gene, Community: Reproductive Technologies among Jewish Israelis
Edited by Daphna Birenbaum-Carmeli and Yoram S. Carmeli

Volume 20
Abortion in Asia: Local Dilemmas, Global Politics
Edited by Andrea Whittaker

Volume 21
Unsafe Motherhood: Mayan Maternal Mortality and Subjectivity in Post-War Guatemala
Nicole S. Berry

Volume 22
Fatness and the Maternal Body: Women's Experiences of Corporeality and the Shaping of Social Policy
Edited by Maya Unnithan-Kumar and Soraya Tremayne

Volume 23
Islam and Assisted Reproductive Technologies: Sunni and Shia Perspectives
Edited by Marcia C. Inhorn and Soraya Tremayne

Volume 24
Militant Lactivism?: Attachment Parenting and Intensive Motherhood in the UK and France
Charlotte Faircloth

Volume 25
Pregnancy in Practice: Expectation and Experience in the Contemporary US
Sallie Han

Volume 26
Nighttime Breastfeeding: An American Cultural Dilemma
Cecília Tomori

Volume 27
Globalized Fatherhood
Edited by Marcia C. Inhorn, Wendy Chavkin and José-Alberto Navarro

Volume 28
Cousin Marriages: Between Tradition, Genetic Risk and Cultural Change
Edited by Alison Shaw and Aviad Raz

Volume 29
Achieving Procreation: Childlessness and IVF in Turkey
Merve Demircioğlu Göknar

ACHIEVING PROCREATION
Childlessness and IVF in Turkey

Merve Demircioğlu Göknar

berghahn
NEW YORK • OXFORD
www.berghahnbooks.com

First published in 2015 by

Berghahn Books

www.BerghahnBooks.com

Library of Congress Cataloging-in-Publication Data

Göknar, Merve Demircioğlu.
Achieving procreation: childlessness and IVF in Turkey / Merve Demircioğlu Göknar.
pages cm. -- (Fertility, reproduction and sexuality; volume 29)
Includes bibliographical references.
ISBN 978-1-78238-634-6 (hardback: alk. paper) -- ISBN 978-1-78238-635-3 (ebook)
1. Childlessness--Turkey. 2. Infertility--Social aspects--Turkey. 3. Human reproductive technology--Social aspects--Turkey. 4. Social medicine--Turkey. I. Title.
HQ762.T9G65 2015
306.87--dc23

2014039959

British Library Cataloguing in Publication Data

A catalogue record for this book is available from the British Library.

ISBN 978-1-78238-634-6 (hardback)
EISBN 978-1-78238-635-3 (ebook)

To my parents, Sevim and Celil Demircioğlu

Contents

Preface

In vitro fertilization (henceforth IVF) remains a popular hope-engendering procedure for those with fertility issues. As the procedure has become more readily available in Turkey in recent decades, it has found popularity as a news media topic. This, coupled with my decision to research the topic as the focus of my academic career, resulted in many new realizations entering into my awareness. As I learned more about new reproductive technologies and IVF, I was astounded to see the vast numbers of childless couples in fertility clinics. I gleaned new insight into the extent to which people will go in order to have a child. I found that infertility had a negative stigma attached to it. I learned that it ended some marriages and strengthened others. I discovered that for some it ruined their life expectations. Gendered implications also came to light. For instance, the challenges it posed on masculinity or sexual identity for men, or the stress on kin relationships for women were real dynamics for the childless. And yet some women triumphed: despite many emotional and social obstacles, these women could persevere, maintain hope, pursue their goal of motherhood and emerge from this challenge with increased self-confidence and faith, and even a child.

In Turkey the media became saturated with the subject of IVF. There were news stories about its success as well as about unethical IVF physicians who engaged in fraud (e.g. those who used sperm other than the husband's in order to increase the success rate). Informative articles in newspapers and discussion programs on television abounded. Some television shows even gave away IVF treatments as prizes. On those programmes, I witnessed the social outcomes of being childless. On one such television programme (the Seda Sayan Show on channel Kanal D), the host would regularly read letters faxed to her by people who demanded the gratis

IVF treatments she offered on the show. Some of these childless women had written dramatic accounts of their life stories: ruined relationships with female affines, the possibility of divorce (or a second wife) and the challenges one had to endure as a childless woman. These letters revealed that childlessness was not only a personal frustration due to not meeting a life ideal, but also a social challenge that childless women had to face daily.

This was my first encounter with the social impacts of infertility. I was a single woman in my late twenties at the time, completing a master's degree in anthropology. Personally, I was ambivalent about having children one day. I had lived in Istanbul among well-educated, career-driven people. Family was important to the people I knew, but most of my girlfriends had prioritized their careers. I had only one friend who had a child at the time. None of my friends spoke negatively of childless married couples. Within such a social milieu, I remained oblivious to the social challenges of infertility.

In Turkey, next to childlessness, not having a son is considered by many a tragic situation. I was more familiar with this dynamic in my own life. My father never made peace with the reality of not having a son. Although he has been a loving and caring father all my life, he has grieved over this. This sentiment is the closest I could get to the experience of childlessness up until this time in my life.

The media coverage of IVF and its growing popularity in Turkey sparked my curiosity about the social impacts of childlessness. During my research about IVF and infertility, the popularity of IVF in Turkey peaked, yet the challenges of being childless remained unknown to many. Against such turmoil of media coverage about IVF, one had to ask: why do people opt for IVF (or choose not to)? What is it like to remain childless in such a pronatalist context? What does it mean to be infertile? Why do people want to have children or to become parents? From within the context of these questions was the genesis of my desire to examine assisted reproductive technologies and IVF.

Acknowledgements

Embarking on fieldwork and writing up a monograph is often a lonely and challenging experience. It requires one to maintain internal motivation while also relying on a community of colleagues, mentors, friends and family. Therefore I owe the following persons my gratitude for supporting me in accomplishing this work. I would like to express my deepest gratitude to Dame Prof. Marilyn Strathern for her encouragement and support. Her distinguished position in the field of social anthropology has been inspirational, and has allowed me access to invaluable intellectual guidance.

The research for this book was made available by the following funding opportunities: British Council Chevening and TEV (Turkish Education Foundation) Joint Scholarship, Evans Funds and Richards Fund (both made available by the Department of Social Anthropology at the University of Cambridge), William Wyse Studentship, Wyse Research Fund and Wyse 4th Year Funding (available through Trinity College and the Department of Social Anthropology at the University of Cambridge), Cambridge University Overseas Research Trust and Trinity Hall Studentship. I am immensely grateful to all of these funding bodies.

I wish to thank Dr Yael Navaro-Yashin, Prof. Jeanette Edwards and Dr Morgan Clarke for their time in relaying insightful suggestions and commentary on early versions of the book. I wish to express my gratitude to Prof. Akile Gürsoy and Dr Oktay Duran who have always been greatly supportive of my academic career.

I am eternally grateful to the following people: Hacer Karaman, Kahraman Karaman, Banu Karaman Menemencioğlu, Hasibe Kılıç, Filiz İsfendiyaroğlu, Lal İsfendiyaroğlu and Dr Aytuğ Kolankaya. Throughout my fieldwork and in the course of writing the book they were my greatest source of support.

Words cannot express my thanks to my lovely aunt Sabire Abdik, who passed away a few months before I completed writing. Her encouragement provided me with patience and hope whenever I lost them.

I am lucky to have met the most wonderful people during this research. I am obliged to İİdil and her lovely parents Elif and Osman and her aunt Selin who welcomed me as a member of their family and who did their best to support my research. I wish to thank to all the women in the villages, in the IVF clinics and at other locations as well who generously shared their precious time with me, revealing their most personal experiences. Among them I owe special thanks to Kerime who became a precious source of support for me. I am grateful to all the physicians and staff at both of the IVF clinics for their hospitality and efforts to facilitate my research. I am immensely thankful to the owner of the North Clinic and the director of the South Clinic. These people enabled my research in the two clinics by granting me access to their facilities. Their names remain undisclosed in order to respect the privacy of the clinics.

I am indebted to my husband Evren Göknar who was the utmost source of help and inspiration during the writing-up process of the book. He dedicated endless hours to editing my writing, and enriched my arguments with perceptive comments. I am also thankful to my dear son Milas whose second year of life coincided with the last year of revising this book. His easygoing and happy character made completing this project much easier than expected.

I would like to thank my dear sister Müge Ersin who has always supported me during my academic career and before. She is such a remarkable person in terms of encouraging and helping.

Finally, I owe my thanks to my parents to whom I dedicate this book. My mother Sevim Demircioğlu and my father Celil Demircioğlu are exceptional people whom I proudly take as role models. Throughout my entire life they have helped me in every imaginable way.

I would also dedicate this book to those who have found it difficult or impossible to: conceive, become parents, attain the life of their dreams, be accepted as complete adults in their communities, be taken seriously, fulfil life's purpose, actualize their gendered roles, love (themselves) or be loved by others.

INTRODUCTION

This book explores the dynamics that inform the demand for in vitro fertilization in Turkey. To this end, I examine women's experiences of childlessness and the greater conceptual significance of children in their lives. I explore the influence of social relationships on childless lives. I focus on the experience of childless women before they start the treatment, rather than during or after the treatment.

The research was conducted in the northwestern part of Turkey. The first part of the research was undertaken in two IVF clinics, in Istanbul and in the outskirts of Istanbul. I interviewed women undergoing IVF (133 interviews in total ranging from a few minutes to two hours) as well as the medical IVF staff. The second part of the research took place in two villages about three hours by car from Istanbul. In the villages I had the chance to observe the implications of childlessness in the context of social relations.

Infertility and Assisted Reproductive Technologies

The definition of infertility is ambiguous (Sandelowski 1993: 55) if not self-imposed (Pfeffer 1987: 83). Infertility had at one point been defined by the WHO (World Health Organization) as 'the inability to conceive within two years of exposure to pregnancy'.[1] In November 2009, the WHO altered this definition, and in *The Revised Glossary for Assisted Reproduction Technology (ART) Terminology*, recognized infertility as a 'disease':[2]

> Infertility (clinical definition): a disease of the reproductive system defined by the failure to achieve a clinical pregnancy after twelve months or more of regular unprotected sexual intercourse.

As the WHO also makes explicit this time, the definition is a clinical one. It is predicated upon biological incapability, and so falls short of acknowledging a whole range of critical issues that derive from the social experience of being infertile, as my research shows, as does other research on infertility in Egypt (Inhorn 1994, 1996), in Lebanon (Inhorn 2004, 2006b, Clarke 2008, 2009), in Israel (Birenbaum-Carmeli and Carmeli 2010, Birenbaum-Carmeli and Inhorn 2011, Haelyon 2006, Inhorn and Birenbaum-Carmeli 2009a, 2009b, Kahn 2000, Soffer and Birenbaum-Carmeli 2010), in Iran (Tremayne 2006) and in India (Riessman 2000a, 2000b) as well as in Turkey (Gürtin 2009, 2012a), among others.

In Turkish, *kısır* means infertile or barren. For many people it is a humiliating word. I have encountered the word sixteen times among 133 interviews. Only two childless women used the word to describe themselves. For some people, only permanent reproductive incapacity may imply infertility. Couples who pursue IVF may not consider themselves infertile, for they still have a chance to conceive, whereas others may consider anyone who seeks a cure from IVF to be infertile.

Infertility has a variety of implications for couples. The gender identities of men and women can be contested due to infertility. For some, childlessness may also connote unrealized life goals, or a life of emotional suffering. However, in stark contrast, some couples in my research consider infertility to be a test given by God, and thus welcome the opportunity to prove one's faith in God's will (as also seen in Inhorn's research with the urban, poor infertile women in Egypt, 1996).

Infertility has been approached from a variety of perspectives in anthropological literature. The influence of religion on the conception of infertility and on the treatment of infertile people is one of them. Religious beliefs can inform the interpretation and experience of infertility that may lead to social exclusion of the infertile woman (N. Price 1998), denial of after-death rituals (Ebin 1994), or aggravation of the stigma based on promotion of motherhood (Inhorn 1996: 83, Kahn 2000). In Islamic countries, having children is also seen as a religious duty, whilst motherhood is sacred by nature (Inhorn 1996). Clarke (2008, 2009), Inhorn (1996, 2003a), Kahn (2000) and Tremayne (2006) reveal the ways in which religion can inform the discourses and practices related to IVF in ethnographies from the Middle East. A critical evaluation of religious discourses (and the pertinent literature) in the context of this research will be provided in the second chapter of this book.

Ethnographies of infertility emphasize stereotyping related to infertility. Selfishness is one of the stereotypes about childless women that I have encountered in my research. Infertility may signify misfortune (Feldman-Savelsberg 2002 on the Bangangté of Cameroon, Neff 1994 on the Nayars in South India), sometimes caused by witchcraft, envy or the evil eye (Inhorn 1996 on Egypt, Mitchell and Georges 2000 on Greece) or misfortune as God's will (Thiessen 1999 on Skopska Crna Gora, Macedonia, Inhorn 1996 on Egypt). There is no uniform way of looking at infertility as misfortune in Turkey, where it is possible to perceive infertility both as misfortune given by God and misfortune due to envy or the evil eye.

Metaphors about infertile people also offer insights as to how infertility is interpreted. A metaphor for the infertile may connote uselessness, a waste of resources and failure to realize the aim of life. A childless woman can also be called 'an empty basket' among the Lazi in Turkey (Beller-Hann 1999, Beller-Hann and Hann 2001),[3] a cow which does not give milk or calves (Inhorn 1996: 59) or a tree that does not bear fruit in Egypt (Inhorn 1994, 1996). As I discuss in the next chapter, a childless woman in Turkey can also be referred to as a fruitless tree.

In this book, I will use the term assisted reproductive technologies (henceforth ART). Turkish terms are: *yardımcı üreme teknolojileri* (assisted reproductive technologies) or üremeye *yardımcı tedavi metodları* (treatment methods for assisted reproduction). The use of acronyms for ART is not common in Turkey except in legal documents.

Just a few years since the completion of my research, IVF is no longer perceived as a novel technology. As I discuss below, IVF has gone through a normalization process, which may have increased its acceptance while decreasing its popularity in the media. It does not engender the type of questions and concerns that it had before. During my research, IVF-related news appeared on television almost every day and one newspaper had a daily corner about IVF. After a few years, herbal healing became a more popular topic, as IVF experts were replaced by experts in herbal healing and nutrition. Newspapers followed the same trend as well.

The people I met in the IVF clinics and the two villages where I conducted research used the term *tüp bebek* (test-tube baby) to refer to IVF, as is common throughout Turkey. Everyone I met in the IVF clinics including the medical personnel and the interviewees used the terms 'sperm' and *yumurta* (egg) to refer to gametes. In the villages I saw that the media popularity of IVF had familiarized people with 'sperm' and *yumurta* as essential components for conceiving a baby. To refer to sperm, the word *döl* was sometimes used as well as 'sperm'. They used *yumurta* in reference to ova.

In vitro fertilization (IVF) refers, in brief, to any assisted reproduction treatment that involves the conception of sperm and ova outside the body (as opposed to *in vivo*, in the body). This is so concise a definition that it is inevitably misleading. I provide a summary of the procedure below to give an idea of how much is obscured in this definition.

The IVF Process in Brief

In the first stage of the process, there is an introductory meeting (ön *görüşme*) with the IVF physician,[4] where a couple learns about the treatment and the clinic, and the physician learns about the couple's reproductive history (involving when they first tried to conceive and what happened after that, including all the treatments undergone and tests taken), habits such as smoking, and the start date of the next menstrual period.

A variety of drugs are used in IVF treatment, along with two 'protocols' (short and long). The preference for a protocol is made mainly depending on the age of the patient. Most of the treatments I observed were long protocols, which lasted about three weeks. The short protocol, which involves intensive hormone intake over ten days, is preferred for women who are forty years old and more. The process I describe here reflects the long protocol. During the treatment, women attend the clinic about 4–5 times for monitoring (*takip*), once for oocyte retrieval and once for embryo transfer within three weeks. The treatment from the first day of using drugs to the day of the pregnancy test is called a 'cycle' in the medical terminology. In Turkish, this word is *siklus*, but its use is limited to medical professionals.

The first part of the cycle is called 'superovulation (follicular stimulation) and monitoring'. A female body has two ovaries and in each ovary (*yumurtalık*) there are follicles, each of which contains one oocyte (egg, *yumurta*). Normally a number of follicles start growing each month but only one of them reaches the mature stage and releases its oocyte (ovulation). With superovulation, the development of several mature follicles is intended.

Superovulation has two phases. The first is called 'down regulation' (*hormonların baskılanması*) and the second is 'stimulation' (*hormonların uyarılması*). During the down regulation, women are given GnRH (gonadotropin-releasing hormone) analogues in order to prevent the ovarian production of endogenous hormones that can interfere with the production of follicles. This drug is taken every day by injection or nasal spray. Depending on the type of drugs used, women have intramuscular injections or they administer the injections themselves subcutaneously two fingers below their belly button using an auto-injector. During this phase it is important that ovaries are kept inactive. To check this, women undergo a vaginal ultrasound about 12–14 days later.

During the stimulation (or monitoring) phase, which lasts 10–12 days, women also inject themselves with drugs containing FSH (follicle-stimulating hormone) and LH (luteinizing hormone) every day in order to stimulate the production of several follicles. They decrease the dose of the GnRH analogue, but continue to inject it daily. Thus, women may have to administer injections to themselves twice or three times a day during this period. During this phase women go to the IVF centre every other day to monitor the growth of their follicles.

When the follicle size and oestrogen levels are ideal, the next step is the final maturation of the follicles. Women stop the injections they have been taking so far. They are given a different injection, of human chorionic gonadotropin (hCG).

After 34–36 hours, couples visit the IVF centre for the oocyte retrieval operation and semen collection. Oocytes are aspirated from follicles through the vagina with ultrasound guidance while women are under sedation. Oocyte retrieval lasts about twenty minutes and women rest for thirty minutes to two hours after the procedure. Women sometimes experience abdominal or pelvic pain. Men provide a sample of semen by masturbation at this time. Embryologists clear the sperm from the semen, and the oocyte from the follicular liquid. They perform tests on the sperm to choose the fastest ones with normal shape and movement.

In conventional IVF, which is almost never employed in Turkey any more, a few thousand sperm with one oocyte are placed in a petri dish in a culture medium – hence the name *in vitro*, meaning 'in glass'. Fertilization is expected within eighteen hours.

An alternative technique is Intracytoplasmic Sperm Injection (ICSI), in which each oocyte is injected with a single sperm by an embryologist. This technique, which has turned out to be a great advantage in male infertility cases, has widely replaced conventional IVF in Turkey. This is mainly because IVF clinics, which want a high rate of 'success', want a lower risk, and so prefer that at least the penetration of the egg be guaranteed.

Couples are informed about the fertilization the day after the oocyte retrieval. The embryo transfer is made usually on the second or third day after the oocyte retrieval (these days, blastocyst transfer on the fifth day is also widespread). Embryo transfer does not require sedation for women who are able to undergo gynaecological examination. In Turkey, the maximum number of embryos that can be transferred is now one (at the time of the research it was three). Twelve days after the embryo transfer, a pregnancy test – measuring the BHCG (beta human chorionic gonadotropin level) in blood – is performed.

The summary given here is still too succinct to give an overall picture of the IVF treatment. The process from the beginning to the end can vary according to the drugs and methods used, health complications experienced and possible failures at each stage. Fear and frustration, as well as hope and joy, are also part of the treatment for many.

IVF in Turkey

Since the birth of Louise Brown, the first IVF baby in 1978, four million IVF babies have been born worldwide (Russell 2010). IVF arrived in Turkey in 1987 and the number of IVF centres in Turkey significantly increased in one decade, from twenty-two in 1998 to ninety-three in 2008.[5] The Turkish Ministry of Health does not disclose any statistics regarding IVF to the public (except the names of active IVF clinics). The ministry refused to answer my questions regarding the number of IVF cycles and the number of IVF babies born to date. The only information they did provide me with was the yearly growth of the number of IVF centres in Turkey. According to a newspaper article (Çelebi 2011), it is estimated that over 50,000 IVF babies have been born in Turkey, and Turkey is the seventh country in terms of the number of IVF treatments performed after Israel, France, Spain, the United Kingdom, the United States and Germany. The total number of IVF cycles per year is over 40,000. However, the article mentions that according to Bahçeci, a well-known IVF specialist in Turkey, there are 500,000 people who are in need of IVF, a statistic that indicates that state financial support for IVF is insufficient (just one of several reasons for not opting for IVF, which this book elucidates).

In Turkey, IVF is available only to heterosexual married couples. Third-party assisted reproduction treatment is illegal. Unlike for the Shia Muslims in Iran and Lebanon (Clarke 2006a, b, 2007 a–d, 2008, 2009, Inhorn 2004, 2006b, Tremayne 2006), gamete (sperm or ova) donation and surrogacy are not possible in most of the Sunni Muslim world. The Turkish Republic of Northern Cyprus is a notable exception and is preferred by Turkish couples who seek IVF via donated ova, sperm, embryo or surrogacy. Greece and Israel are among the other favourite destinations for 'reproductive tourism'.[6] Turkish law permits freezing embryos for five years with the consent of both spouses. In the case of death of a spouse, frozen embryos are destroyed.[7]

The latest legislation in Turkey, as of 6 March 2010 brought enormous changes regarding the use of ART. Now not only the practice of IVF using donor gametes or embryos is illegal, but even referring patients to such practices abroad, or informing patients about such treatments is not allowed anymore (Gürtin 2010, 2011). The head of South Clinic (pseudonym) where I did research told me that he would not even mention a word to anyone about those practices anymore, now that it could be considered a criminal act. An IVF clinic can be shut down for three months if any IVF physician is found to refer couples to donor IVF (a second occurrence of such an act can result in the total termination of the clinic). All people involved in such acts including physicians, gamete/embryo recipients and gamete/embryo donors are prosecuted. I hope the later parts of this introduction on the government's strong support for the ideology of the 'sacred family' will make the incentives for such legislation a bit more understandable. However, this is not to say that the reasons underlying such forceful laws are understood or approved by the thousands who are in need of donor gametes or embryos.

Another major change in the practice of IVF in Turkey, brought about by the same legislation, is about the number of embryos that can be transferred to a woman's womb. During the time of my research, it was possible to carry out embryo transfer with up to three embryos. For those who had a history of failed IVF cycles or who were above thirty-nine years old, four embryos could be transferred.[8] This new legislation introduces the practice of 'single embryo transfer' (SET) to Turkey. The transfer of only one embryo is allowed for women under the age of 35 for the first two cycles. Women under 35 who have had two failed cycles of IVF and women above 34 – in each cycle – can undergo IVF with a maximum of two embryos. This law is justified with the increased health risks associated with multiple pregnancies. Since the legislation came into force long after this research took place, the book will not reflect on the current laws.

Married women must be over twenty-three and under forty years old in order to be eligible for funding via the state's social security institutions,[9] they should have been insured for at least five years by one of those social security institutions, and should have failed to conceive for three years. Childless couples who meet these conditions can get a medical report from a teaching or research hospital.[10] The cost of treatment at the time the research took place (depending on the quantity of drugs a woman needed, as well as on the clinic) was around 3,000–4,000 U.S. dollars or 5,000–6,000 Turkish liras, including the drugs. In a teaching or research hospital, a couple with a medical report (mentioned above) could have treatment for as little as 410 Turkish liras and pay half the cost of the medicine (for two cycles of IVF).

Mass media was the medium through which 'truths' about IVF were generated during my research. IVF was known to everyone, but there were alternative truth claims for IVF. Many people assumed that IVF was implemented with the sperm of a third party. This was because of the sporadic appearance of news in the mass media about the illegal use of third-party sperm in IVF or artificial insemination (with or without the knowledge of the couples).[11] Paternal relatedness in these narratives was reckoned genetically, and the man whose wife underwent IVF was suspected of not being the 'real father' of the IVF child.

During this research, a newspaper (*Posta*) had a daily corner about IVF. Television programmes had IVF specialists who provided information about the treatment. Sometimes religious specialists, nutrition experts and celebrities joined these discussions. All of these people contributed to the formation of discursive truths about infertility, IVF and motherhood. For example, IVF specialists stressed that 'men, too can be infertile', nutritionists underscored that 'overweight people have problems related to fertility', while religious specialists warned against 'committing a sin by having a child in unconventional ways' (such as surrogacy). Celebrities making claims about adoption as a more 'appropriate' solution (compared to IVF) for having a child marginalized certain treatments and the people who underwent them.

Some of these programmes also featured members of the public. For example, one daily programme hosted about a hundred guests who went to watch the show and take advantage of the gifts distributed on the programme.[12] These gifts ranged from household appliances and furniture to funding for an IVF cycle. Another daily programme sponsored unlimited cycles of IVF for women.[13] IVF emerged as a pop culture artefact during my research that attracted popular attention, was distributed as a postmodern gift, and which created a gamut of truth claims about the people who underwent it. Childless women participated in creating these truths by narrating their childless lives and by representing a needy self to convince the programme hosts to give them the 'gift'. As a pop culture artefact, the popularity of IVF in the media later diminished, despite its enduring significance for millions of childless couples and their families.

During this research there was a television series called *Bebeğim* (My Baby) about a woman who had a child via surrogacy.[14] This series precipitated a debate in the media by journalists, sociologists and viewers of the series. The fact that surrogacy is a reality in Turkey despite its illegality and controversial image became apparent in daily television shows, in which couples who commissioned surrogates as well as surrogate mothers participated. Discourses about the 'natural desire' and 'natural need' for motherhood as well as the 'natural way' (or appropriate ways) to be a mother were repeatedly reproduced in discussions pertinent to IVF.

An interesting aspect of these appearances of IVF in the media and of the discussions that took place around them was the normalization of IVF (Thompson 1998, 2005: 79–115). Childless couples participated in this normalization. A woman could ask for a sofa along with IVF as a gift in these programmes. Infertility, once always concealed (and still concealed by many), could be normalized in a Foucauldian manner via medicalization, by defining it as a disease, or by presenting it as a financial problem compared to the lack of money to buy a sofa.[15]

While infertility is medicalized, IVF is socialized. For example, the fact that the practice of polygyny[16] has diminished due to the increasing use of IVF is a recurrent discourse in newspaper articles, including the internet and religious newspapers. First, this discourse presents polygyny as a social problem. Then the claim that men who can now have a child via IVF do not need a second wife (*kuma*: concubine) presents IVF as a solution to this social problem. Another common narrative in news articles about IVF is the presentation of childlessness and of not having a son as social problems, and the presentation of IVF as a solution to these problems.

In these newspaper articles, claims that polygyny was the cultural solution to childlessness or not having a son before IVF make reference to a specific region in Turkey: the 'southeastern' part. In these articles, it is the southeastern (or eastern) region where husbands take a second wife (*kuma*) when they do not have a son, and it is women from the east/southeast, who do not want a *kuma* in their homes, who subsequently fill up IVF clinics. This narrative, by localizing childlessness or sonlessness[17] and its allegedly inevitable consequence, polygyny (taking a *kuma*), essentializes the 'culture' of people of a certain place and also normalizes IVF.

De Kok (2009: 211) warns against the normalization of certain practices as 'cultural' by people who want to legitimate them. Based on his research on opinions of infertility in Malawi during 2002–2003, he shows how:

> respondents account for responses to infertility, such as engaging in extramarital affairs or polygamy, by mobilizing a cultural norm according to which bearing children is expected or required. These accounts construct the aforementioned practices as reasonable, practical solutions for fertility problems, and as scripted, that is, widespread and recurrent. Consequently, respondents normalize practices and play down people's accountability for them.

The Turkish media, in a similar vein, normalizes polygyny in the context of the southeast part of Turkey, but cannot normalize it for others for whom polygyny is considered a social problem. The narrative of before and after the advent of IVF resolves this conflict. Before the advent of IVF, polygyny is justified with reference to having a son as the 'cultural norm' (but only in the 'southeastern culture'), while after the arrival of IVF, pursuing IVF is normal (still in the context of those cultural norms that compel one to have children or specifically sons).

Another newspaper article about surrogacy appeared amidst the discussions triggered by the television serial, *Bebeğim*, mentioned above. Okyay, the consultant on the film, commented upon surrogacy:

> Turkish society is already open to this topic and ready for it. Because especially in Anatolia, when the fertility of a woman is not considered enough, the problem is solved by a *kuma* (a second wife via religious marriage). Furthermore, the babies born to the *kuma* are registered as the children of the wife who is married to the man with a civil marriage. In the serial, this problem is solved by finding a surrogate and getting pregnant with IVF.[18]

For Okyay, Turkey is ready for surrogacy, which has similarities to polygyny (already practised by some people in Turkey). This association of established cultural practices with new ones provides a creative way to normalize a practice such as surrogacy. By 'piggybacking' surrogacy onto polygyny, surrogacy also becomes culturized.

Literature on IVF and Infertility in Turkey

In anthropological literature around the world, IVF has created debates on a variety of critical issues, ranging from unequal access to the treatment, to the bioethical or biopolitical considerations with regards to its use, objectification of the female body, commoditization of body parts in the form of gametes, reproductive tourism, transfer of technologies (and ideologies) to different cultures and the status of the woman versus the embryo. It has raised concerns over the ideology of the sacred family in religious or state ideologies.

The Humboldt University carried out a collaborative research project in Germany and Turkey to investigate the implications of ART and adoption on kinship, entitled 'Kinship as Representation of Social Order and Practice: Knowledge, Performativity and Legal-Ethical Regulation'. It was a long-term project conducted during 2004–2012. The results of the research can be found in an edited collection, *Reproductive Technologies in Global Form* (Knecht, Klotz and Beck 2012).

Gürtin conducted comparative research on IVF in Turkey and England within IVF clinics during 2006–2007 for her PhD dissertation at the Centre for Family Research, University of Cambridge, entitled 'The ART of Making Babies: Social Constructions of Turkish IVF'. She conducted interviews with patients, practitioners and experts, both inside and outside clinics. Her interest lies more in the experience of IVF and third-party IVF. By comparison, this book is focused on the pre-IVF experience of infertility.[19] Gürtin (2009) also provides an account of Turkish immigrant women's experiences of childlessness and IVF in London.[20]

In addition, a recent medical journal article investigates public opinion on oocyte donation in Turkey (Işıkoğlu et al. 2006). It is the first investigation into the topic to be conducted in a secular Muslim country. The data from four hundred interviews with women and men in rural and urban districts of Antalya (a large city on the Mediterranean coast) shows that most of the participants did not have objections to oocyte donation. Only fifteen per cent totally objected (It would be useful to know the same population's response to the use of donor sperm). This positive attitude towards oocyte donation in Antalya, however, should not be taken as representative of Turkey. Another study (Baykal et al. 2008) examines the opinions of infertile Turkish women on gamete donation and surrogacy. 23.1 and 15.1 per cent of the respondents of the study would accept oocyte donation and surrogacy respectively if they needed (the acceptance rate for sperm donation is only 3.4 per cent).

Research has also been done on the psychiatric implications of infertility. Özkan and Baysal's (2006) research with fifty infertile and forty fertile women revealed that infertile women, especially the ones with lower rates of employment, education and economic status and longer experience with infertility, suffered severely from depression.

IVF is also becoming a prominent theme for popular non-academic books in Turkey. There are now two books published by medical experts as guidance for women who want to pursue IVF (Bahçeci and Aktan 2007, Gülekli 2006), a book written by a journalist – again as a guidebook – who went through the treatment herself (Aydın 2009), a novel about a woman who undergoes IVF with sperm from her fiancé who is in a coma (Kefeli 2008), as well as a book about the Koran's view of IVF (Duman 1991).

It is important to note that despite the pivotal place of children in Turkey, and despite the significant ramifications of childlessness (on women, men and families), there has not been much anthropological interest in the issue of not having a child. The patrilocally extended family versus nuclear family type was once a source of interest for sociological and anthropological accounts of the family. The patriarchal structures inherent in virilocal households and the contemporary changes in those structures were often analysed (Duben 1982, Ilcan 1994b, 1996, Kağıtçıbaşı 1982b, 1982c, Rasuly-Paleczek 1996, Vergin 1985). Regarding kinship and gender, marriage practices have also been explored (Bates 1974, Hart 2007, Ilcan 1994a, 1994b, 1996, Kudat 1974). Gender is often investigated through the framework of patriarchal relationships in the household. Ethnographic accounts tangentially touch on infertility as an unfortunate circumstance for women. Since patriarchy remains the focus for most anthropological research, the failure to have a son has raised more interest. In a similar vein, kinship has been analysed in terms of the significance of having a son in the negotiations for patriarchal power (e.g. Delaney 1991, Ilcan 1996, Stirling 1965: 42, White 1994). This is the first anthropological manuscript on Turkey with regards to infertility and ART.

Places and Persons

Defining the field site is a matter of scale and choice. Because of its geography, history and varied cultural influences, it remains difficult to determine whether Turkey is part of the Middle East the Mediterranean or both. It can also be considered European, Western, non-Western or an amalgam of them all. These field site decisions matter because they inform our theoretical frameworks. Bonaccorso's (2009: xvii) objection to the boundaries of 'Euro-America' (which indicates the discourses relevant to North America and Northern Europe) and Italy's place in relation to it is a case in point. Italy, as a southern European country, is outside the theoretical field of 'Euro-America'. However, Bonaccorso's discussion of kinship reveals important similarities between her field site and 'Euro-American' discourses about the implications of assisted reproductive technologies on kinship.[21]

The reasons behind conducting this research in Turkey were based on its contrast to the broader fields in which Turkey is found. Primarily, Turkey has a distinct place in the Middle East for being the only country with an Islamic population that has a secular civil constitution, and powerful religious authorities (such as the *ulema* or *mullahs* in Iran or Lebanon) do not exist.[22] On the other hand, the state is not totally independent of religious influence. The laws pertaining to assisted reproductive technologies are consistent with the opinions and suggestions of the Presidency of Religious Affairs (*Diyanet İşleri Başkanlığı*). As such, there is 'harmony between secular legislation and religious opinion' (Gürtin 2012a: 286). Among Turkish people there is a growing tendency towards Islamism or at least towards more conservatism, but secularism, the founding ideology of the Turkish Republic, is still reflected in the lives of many Turks. Between the two extremes – from the most secularist to the Islamists, a range of discourses and practices regarding infertility and IVF exists, informed by a range of values, lifestyles and ideologies. As Gürtin (2012a: 286) states, 'as a staunchly secular nation with a Muslim population, as well as a country with great regional variation and enormous socioeconomic divisions, Turkey often represents paradoxes and hybrids for researchers'.

The majority of Turks are Sunni Muslims (the largest sect of Islam) with a minority of Alevis (a Shia group of Islam of most of whose adherents live in Turkey). Turkey's legislation on IVF reflects the Sunni consensus, which bans third-party gamete donation, surrogacy and limits IVF to married couples only. These prohibitions by the Sunnis aim to protect patrilineage (Inhorn and Tremayne 2012: 5, Clarke 2009). Turkish legislators, despite the similarity of their legislation on ART with that of other Sunni communities, do not accept the influence of religion on legislation. As Gürtin states, they may rather justify this similarity with an explanation based on 'culture' rather than 'religion': 'Although it may not be practically possible to disintegrate "culture" from "religion" within the secular politics of Turkey, the latter is unacceptable as a causal explanation of state regulation, whereas the former can be used to mobilize democratic aspirations' (Gürtin 2012a: 304).

As well as being Middle Eastern, Turkey, as Navaro-Yashin (2002: 9) argues, has always been European. As far as IVF treatment is concerned, the motivation of achievement underpins people's persistence with the procedure, just as in England (Franklin 1997). At the same time, an Islamic Middle Eastern approach also informs the attitude towards conception via IVF: the rhetoric of God's will.[23] Thus Turkey, as an Islamic-European site with similarities to the European and American discourses, proves to be a unique field for the study of infertility and IVF.

The research for this book was undertaken in the northwestern part of Turkey, in Istanbul and a neighbouring city. Doing research in the western part of Turkey was a deliberate choice. Stereotypes of social conditions (especially regarding gender and kinship) exist in the eastern (or southeastern) part of Turkey. Honour crimes, bride price, extreme son preference, and polygyny are among the practices typically attributed to the 'easterners' of Turkey. These practices were indeed more common among the people in my research who hailed from or were living in the east. The importance of having a son was more explicit among them than any other group. But still, these practices are in no way restricted to the people who live in the east, nor are they common to everyone in the east.

Whenever I explained my research topic to a Turk, the same question often followed: 'Why don't you do your research in the east/southeast?' This implied that in the east/southeast, gender inequality was so acute that richer data regarding the suffering of the infertile could be available. I was not after suffering, and if there were any, I would rather show that it was not confined to the east. The question above justified my decision to conduct research in the west. I was never concerned about 'representing Turkey' but I wanted to avoid 'representing the east' while excluding others in Turkey. My research shows that stigma attached to infertility exists and is not confined to the east. It is prevalent in varying degrees and forms among people I have met from all over Turkey. There are many women who suffer from the pressure to have a baby (or even a son) in both Istanbul and in the villages where I did research.

The IVF Clinics

As I have stated above, my ethnography was divided between the observation of IVF clinics and of family life in villages. First I did research in IVF clinics for about six months. I call these IVF clinics the North Clinic, and the South Clinic.[24] The North Clinic is on the European side of Istanbul, in a quarter inhabited by working-class people as well as the wealthy. The South Clinic is located in the outskirts of Istanbul, on the Asian side. Long before any fieldwork took place, while drafting my research proposal, I was able to arrange to visit these two IVF clinics for my research. A family friend owned the hospital where the North Clinic operated, and the head of the South Clinic was a friend of mine. I was welcomed at both clinics, and the IVF physicians were often supportive. There was no unease due to my presence in the clinics – unlike for example Bonaccorso's (2009: 19) research experience in IVF clinics in Milan.

I went to these IVF clinics five days a week, from morning to evening. I conducted interviews with women who were undergoing IVF as well as the IVF physicians. I also had many informal conversations with the physicians, nurses, secretaries and cleaning staff. I recorded the interviews when the women gave permission. Women were interviewed only in privacy, without their partners or others present. There were only a few times when their husbands or mothers attended the interviews, but this was always after an interview with them alone. I sometimes chatted with their kin (including mothers-in-law) in the waiting room. The interviews always took place in Turkish.

The North Clinic was located on the European side of Istanbul, in a district populated mostly with migrants from all over Turkey, as well as from the Balkans. Sixty-four per cent of women were primary school graduates and I met only one university graduate among them. Most of them lived in various parts of Istanbul, while a third of them were living in other parts of Turkey. There was a Turkish woman among the interviewees who came from Germany. The average length of marriage was nine years among the women I interviewed. There were six women married for 17 years. Eighty-five per cent of women were housewives.

The South Clinic was on the outskirts of Istanbul. It was part of a new hospital with imposing modern architecture, which stood in strong contrast to the shanty town surroundings. The hospital was close to an industrial zone, and so factory workers visited the hospital as well as affluent people who wanted access to the latest technology. The IVF unit also had a branch in an elite quarter of Istanbul. However, all the women who underwent IVF there had embryo transfer and oocyte retrieval operations in the central hospital.

In the South Clinic, I had the chance to meet IVF patients of a higher socioeconomic status than in the North Clinic. The number of women who had university level education (38 per cent of women) was greater than the number of women who had only primary school education (31 per cent of women). This was also the case with their husbands. Half of the women were housewives. Five of them came from distant parts of Turkey. The average length of marriage for the women was eight years.

I was not denied access to the women in either clinic. The physicians were never concerned about whom I interviewed. They did not care if women spoke negatively about the treatment. Access was not negotiated based on whom to interview, but on the stage of the process during which I would do the interview.

In the North Clinic, the head of the IVF unit allowed me to talk to the women only at certain stages of the IVF process. In the beginning of the research, I could talk to women only after the initial meeting (*ön görüşme*) with the physician. This was certainly the worst stage for conducting an interview with the women. In their first meetings, they had so many questions on their minds about the treatment, the physician and the clinic that they found it hard to concentrate on my questions. I often felt I was disturbing them when they were looking forward to leaving the clinic and talking to their husbands about their first meetings. After a few weeks I persuaded the physician to let me interview the women at later stages of the process. I could then talk to them at the 'follow-up' (*takip*) stage (this is the superovulation and monitoring stage), but never during the days they had oocyte retrieval or embryo transfer. I was told that the women needed rest instead of discourse for those two days. Still, interviewing women during the later stages of the process proved extremely fruitful for me. The interviews could continue much longer, and the women felt much more comfortable (as did I). At these stages, they had often already seen me a few times in the clinic and sometimes had already spoken to me.

In the South Clinic, the physicians never interfered in the research process. The head of the IVF unit told me that I could talk to anyone I wanted. He suggested that I talk to women on the days of the oocyte retrieval and embryo transfer. On those days, women had plenty of time for the interview since they were waiting for their turn for hours before the operation, and they were resting after the operation. The women were often willing to talk to me, because most of the time they were bored and anxious while waiting.

In addition to the head of the clinic, there was an additional IVF physician in the North Clinic. Both of them were in their forties. In the IVF unit, there was a large waiting room where the reception area was located. The physicians' offices were at one side of the room. The operating room was separated from the waiting room with sliding glass doors. On one side of the doors, there was a small corridor that led to the operating room and recovery room. People who were going to the operating room had to remove their shoes at that corridor and wear flip-flops. There were also blue gowns to put on.

The waiting room was almost always packed with women. Their husbands usually accompanied them for the initial meetings, and during embryo transfer and oocyte retrieval. For other scheduled visits, the women would often visit the clinic alone or with a female relative or friend. Two secretaries and the nurses would gather around the reception table when they had no other work to do. I too would join them and chat when I could not otherwise conduct an interview.

During the first weeks at the North Clinic, the head of the IVF unit used to call me into his room when there was an introductory meeting. He introduced me as a researcher who was interested in hearing why they were there and who had some questions to ask. He encouraged the couples to speak to me. When I started to interview the 'follow-up' patients, the nurses and secretaries became my sources of support. They introduced me to women, and provided me with their brief histories. I sometimes approached women myself, but more often I was introduced to them at the reception desk.

For our interviews, I took women through the glass doors to the corridor leading to the operating room. There were two chairs in that corridor on which we could sit. There was not enough privacy there, since it was possible for noise to pass through the glass doors. Passers-by were also disturbing. However, there was no other place for interviews, since I was not permitted to interview post-operation patients in the recovery room. A few times I interviewed women in the physicians' offices when they were available. The improvement in comfort and privacy was clearly reflected in the depth and length of the interviews.

Since the head of the South Clinic was familiar with social anthropology (he had taken social anthropology classes), he was sympathetic to the research requirements. He did not introduce me to any of the women. Instead, I was given access to the recovery room where I introduced myself, asked for permission from the women, and then conducted the interviews. The recovery room housed six beds aligned into two rows of three. The beds were separated from each other by plastic privacy curtains. I sat on a stool near the beds when I interviewed the women. There was a small plasma TV hanging from the ceiling in front of each bed. The conditions at this IVF unit reflected the 'modernity' of the hospital, as the women described it. This environment was confusing to some of the women who came from remote rural areas. The environment, so different from their everyday experience, enhanced the liminality of their IVF experience. The interview conditions at this clinic were much better compared to the other one, allowing me to do more recorded interviews.

In both clinics, the physicians favoured the vernacular of the couples. For instance, to refer to a menstrual period, they did not use the words *periyod, menstruasyon* or even *regl,* common among the doctors or educated elite, but rather they used the word *adet.* In contrast to the distance (which implicates authority) deliberately created by physicians using medicalized language (Bonaccorso 2009: 79–81), these physicians were inclined towards creating a sense of trust with their patients. A similar attitude by Turkish physicians towards couples seeking IVF was also noted by Gürtin (2012b): 'Many practitioners, dealing with a diverse range of patients, perceptibly varied their choice of words and general demeanour to facilitate a "dialogue" and to enable better communication with each and every type of patient'. In the spirit of disclosure, the physicians were always explicit about the risk of failure. Nonetheless, they also stressed to most couples that IVF was their only option for conceiving a child.

The interactions of the nurses with women undergoing IVF in the North Clinic were also based on creating warm relationships. In the South Clinic, however, nurses could sometimes be impatient or even arrogant. I witnessed two of them giving only brief explanations of the treatment, and occasionally responding to women's questions as if they were not intelligent enough to understand the treatment. These nurses were uncomfortable with me witnessing their unkind treatment of the women.

My interactions with women undergoing IVF were better than I had expected. Since infertility is a delicate topic which people often conceal and which also can be traumatic, I assumed that women would be reluctant to talk to me. Contrary to my expectations,

I was almost always welcomed, and women at various times remarked that talking to me about their experiences and emotions made them feel better. According to the head of the South Clinic, the women (and therefore the physicians) were pleased to have a sympathetic ear: 'It is good for them to be listened to'. Bonaccorso's (2009: 25) experience with women in IVF clinics is very similar to mine:

> [A] part of me is still surprised at the depth and openness with which couples spoke to me, an absolute stranger. But possibly this occurred precisely because I was an absolute stranger, not unlike an encounter on a train. It is not unusual to share very personal life histories with strangers, one can be honest and direct as there are no implications.

The same applies to the interactions I had with the couples. And it was confirmed during unpleasant encounters when I crossed the boundaries of being a stranger, or perhaps even violated the borders, and told a woman, for example, 'my family hails from the place where you live. We are from the same village.' Uneasy looks and silence followed such impertinent remarks from me. It was even uncomfortable when I once told a woman that like her I had also worked as a product manager. This happened during an interview with Ela at the South Clinic, a 37-year-old woman with a career in marketing. I told Ela that I too had worked in marketing for a time. Before I said that, in her eyes, I was a researcher she met in a clinic. The moment I said I had been a product manager was the instant I moved out of that sphere. Where I belonged shifted, along with the woman's presumptions about me. On these occasions, women could no longer count on the privacy of the encounter. These encounters seemed to be confusing and possibly bothersome for the women.

Despite the importance of providing contextual information about the author (e.g. Edwards 2000: 18) as well as the narrator and the interview environment, I do not provide this for each interview in the book due to space limitations.[25] In addition, similar to Bonaccorso (2009), I aim to underline the repeated patterns or discourses in these narratives by providing as many of them as I can.

The Villages

For the second half of my research I stayed in two villages that were near one another. My main reason for continuing the research outside the clinics was to understand the impact of childlessness on social relationships. I had acquired pertinent insight from the interviews, but a village setting afforded me the opportunity to observe how the politics of childlessness emerged in extended families and among close friends.

Inhorn (2003a: 27), who has worked on IVF and infertility in Egypt for almost twenty years, expressed her regret at not having done participant observation outside the clinics, which constrained her study. In anthropological studies on assisted reproductive technologies, research outside IVF clinics is less common. An exception is a study of fertile people outside clinics by Edwards (2000). Clarke's (2009) work in Lebanon derives from ethnography outside IVF clinics, but it was carried out with Islamic authorities and philosophers rather than childless women themselves. Another notable exception is an ethnography by Kahn (2000) concerning infertility and the Rabbinic discourses and practices related to IVF in Israel.

The villages in which I worked were attached to a small coastal town, three hours away from Istanbul by bus, in the northwestern part of Turkey. There was a minibus service to the coastal town from both of the villages every hour. These villages will be called Village Dere (Stream) and Village Tepe (Hill). The house where I lived was on the outskirts of Village Dere and was also about thirty minutes away from Village Tepe on foot. Dere was a hillside village a fifteen minute walk away from the coastal town, which had schools, small retailers, a hospital, post office, banks, parks, cafes, restaurants and such.[26] Tepe was further up the hill, an hour's walk from the same town.

I started research first in Village Dere, which was closer to where I was living. Most of the inhabitants of Dere were native to the region, but some had migrated from northeastern Turkey. A small minority came from eastern Turkey. A few of the families owned large fruit gardens where other villagers could work to earn daily wages. Since this was far from sufficient, sons were moving out of the village to find jobs elsewhere. Daughters usually married out, so when they married, they left the village as well. This is why most of the inhabitants of the village were elderly people with unmarried daughters. This context was valuable for observing the pressure to get married and have children.

In Tepe, most of the inhabitants were bilingual (Turkish and Bosnian). The first settlers of Village Tepe were Muslim Bosniaks (*Boşnak*) who migrated from Bosnia after Bosnia's separation from the Ottoman Empire at the end of the nineteenth century.[27] More than 90 per cent of the households had Bosniak family members.

Cattle raising was the major income-generating activity and most of the families had fruit gardens. Many villagers owned small-scale businesses in the nearby town centre. The inhabitants of Tepe were wealthy enough to afford to live in patrilineally extended houses. It was thus possible to observe the ways in which the relationships in extended families informed the experience of childlessness.

I was living in Dere with the parents of a friend and her aunt. The first reason I chose to stay there was that I had a limited time (six months) and this family would help me meet people and be welcomed in a shorter period of time. I refer to my friend as Idil, and her parents as Elif and Osman in this book. I call her aunt, who also lives in the same house, Selin. Selin spends the whole year there, while the others live there for only half of the year. In winter, Idil's parents go back to their house in Istanbul. All the members of the family did their best to support my research. They answered all of my questions patiently, they introduced me to the people they knew in Village Dere and around it, and they accompanied me on my visits to houses in Dere during the first weeks. Then I decided to continue doing research in Tepe as well, where they hardly knew anyone. Elif and I visited houses together and introduced ourselves. Having Elif with me made my acceptance to the village much easier.

In Tepe, I initially knocked on doors of houses with Elif in an attempt to establish friendships once we were invited in. A Koran course started in the village, which the local women started to attend. This was fortunate because women aged between 27 and 60 were attending this course to learn the Koranic script.[28] In villages usually children take Koran classes in the mosques during summer holidays. Every morning there was a class for children in the mosque of the village's 'middle quarter'. They learned the principles of Islam and memorized *suras* (certain sections of the Koran under separate names). After the children's class, the women's class would take place. There were nine women including Elif and me. Sometimes the number was higher when others came to practise their reading skills. Thanks to the Koran course, I had the chance to improve friendships with the women. The common experience of being classmates together became the foundation of these relationships.

Idil had been married for four years during my research and she was voluntarily childless. For the people in Dere and Tepe, voluntary childlessness at thirty years old was not easily comprehensible. When Idil was around, I had the chance to observe people's reactions to childlessness as well as the pressure she was encountering from family and friends.

I always spoke in Turkish in both of the villages. Elderly people in Tepe always speak to each other in Bosnian (*Boşnakça*), but in my presence they spoke Turkish, too. Unlike in Village Dere, there were people who were involuntarily childless (five women) in Tepe. This facilitated my research to a large extent by giving me the chance to observe the lives and relationships of childless women. I got close to one of these childless women (Kerime).

There were no schools in Dere, which was closer to the town; students could easily get to school in the nearby town on school buses. There was one mosque. In Tepe there were three mosques, one in each *mahalle* (quarter or neighbourhood), and one primary school (in the whole village) for primary education until the fourth grade. In both villages there were both girls and boys who were receiving university education in various cities in Turkey from Edirne to Istanbul and Izmir.

Both villages were divided into quarters, with names. In Tepe, since it was a larger village, quarters were more important in terms of people's social lives. The closest friendships were within the same quarters. The people I became close to were all living in the same quarter, the 'middle quarter' (*orta mahalle*). There was also an 'upper quarter' (*yukarı mahalle*) and a 'lower quarter' (*aşağı mahalle*).

Life in the two villages was very similar. In both villages, religion remained significant. In both Dere and Tepe the day typically started with practising the morning prayer (*sabah namazı*). Breakfast was followed by domestic and garden chores. Women visited each other in their houses and often did needlework during these visits. In Tepe when they gathered together, they sometimes made *pita börek* otherwise known as *Boşnak böreği* (a kind of pastry common among the Bosniaks, filled with cheese, potatoes or vegetables). In Tepe, women who attended the Koran course also practised reading the Koran together. After dinner, it was common in both villages for families to visit neighbours' houses. If the husbands were not at home, the women would make the visits without them. In both villages, children were sent to Koran classes in the summer to learn about religion. The Bosniak ethnic identity did not seem to have a major influence on the way of life in Village Tepe. Other than the differences specified here (and in Chapter 3 regarding marriage practices), the residents of both villages had similar lifestyles.

Persons

Below is information about the people with whom I developed the closest relationships in the villages, and who consequently appear prominently in this book. There were many houses spread out over a large area on the outskirts of Village Dere in addition to houses inside the quarters of the village. Elif and Selin with whom I was living were always my greatest support; they did their best to help my research in every way. They had strong neighbourhood relationships with a few of the families living on the outskirts of Village Dere. Three of those families in particular became enthusiastic supporters of my research, inviting me every day to their houses in order to 'teach me their way of life'. One of those women, Saadet had a child after sixteen years of marriage. She was over fifty years old and her elder daughter was eighteen years old. She was reluctant to talk about those sixteen years, but she and her husband still shared a lot with me about that time.

Hatice and Yasemin were my dearest friends in Village Dere. They were both single and around thirty years old. Religion was central to Hatice's life. She practised all the compulsory prayers and wore Islamic attire.[29] Her opinions on almost everything were grounded in religion. She often talked about the life of the Prophet and suggested the names of religious books for me to read. Although she wanted to continue school, she had left school at an early age according to her grandmother's wishes. Her twenty-year-old sister Esra was not so pious. She did not wear Islamic attire; indeed, she used to wear knee-length skirts and sleeveless shirts. She was studying media at a university in Izmir, a metropolitan city on the west coast of Turkey. Yasemin's sister, who was getting married to Hatice's brother, was a pious practising Muslim like Hatice. Yasemin did not wear Islamic attire, and she pursued a comparatively independent life. On weekdays she stayed in a town close by (forty-five minutes by car) where she was working. Hatice and Yasemin were close friends and they both cemented a friendship with me.

Kerime's name appears frequently in the book. A 37-year-old involuntarily childless woman, Kerime was my closest friend in Village Tepe. She was one of the attendees of the Koran class. She knew how to read the Koran but she was there in order to improve her reading skills.

Kerime was living with her husband and her husband's elder brother. She had been married for twelve years, and had lived with her mother-in-law until her death two years ago. Kerime worked gathering fruit for daily wages, as well as in her own olive garden. Her husband managed a *kahve* (local coffee shop for men) in the village. They could hardly make ends meet. Kerime had been having hormonal treatment for infertility after her mother-in-law's death. Although one of her fallopian tubes was blocked, Kerime seemed reluctant to try IVF, unlike the ambitious women I had met in the IVF clinics. This was partly due to financial reasons, as well as her husband's objection to IVF.

Kerime was a very friendly woman who loved to spend time with friends, including me. We kept in contact after the fieldwork was over, and she still replies to my questions readily and does her best to be of help to me. She and her husband appeared to love each other, and Kerime confirmed this to me when she talked about their relationship.

Cevriye, a lovely 54-year-old woman with three sons and a daughter, was another one of my Koran classmates. Two of her sons were married, one of whom had a child. Her childless son did not want to undergo IVF. Her other son had only one child, which distressed her: 'I tell them to go to a doctor if they have a problem. One child is not enough in this world.' Although she was encouraging her sons to seek treatment, she didn't pressure them. This was obvious, because Cevriye had a very docile, gentle character and her childless daughter-in-law was fond of her. Cevriye had suffered difficulties with her own parents-in-law – with whom she had lived for sixteen years – but she was not authoritarian to her daughters-in-law. She was also very supportive of me and my research.

Throughout the book, my encounters in the field and information about the interviews are sometimes in the debated 'ethnographic present', despite the fact that they happened six years ago.[30] Sometimes they are in the past tense, even though it is at this moment that I am reproducing them in theoretical frameworks unfamiliar to the persons with whom they were produced initially. As Hastrup (1989 n.d.: 28) notes, 'The dialogue was "then", but the discourse is "now". There is no choice of tense' (cited in Strathern 1991a: 48).

The 'field' was not only composed of the IVF clinics and the villages along with the persons I met there. The Turkish television serials I was watching at home, and even chats with my friends and family, had suddenly become a means of observation from the day I arrived in Turkey as a researcher. The place and the persons were the same to an extent, but it was I who was different. I was a part of my field (Hastrup 1990: 46) and have since been 'no longer the same' (1990: 50).

A Brief Literature Overview on Infertility and ART

A summary of the anthropological and sociological studies as well as the feminist literature on infertility and ART is now available from many sources (for example: Bonaccorso 2009: 2–7, Inhorn 2007c: 1–43, Thompson 2005: 51–75, as well as Clarke 2009 on 'new kinship'; Inhorn and Tremayne 2012 on Islam and ART, and Inhorn et al. 2009 for ART and masculinities). Some ethnographies concern women's subjectivities and experiences related to the IVF treatment rather than making a broader evaluation of infertility. The experiences of women who undergo IVF are studied in the works of Becker (1990, 1994, 1997, 2000) and Franklin (mainly 1997, besides 1988, 1990) whose ethnographies are from the United States and England respectively. Following other feminist writers, Franklin aims to dispel doubts over the devastating consequences of IVF. The overwhelming nature of the treatment is emphasized by focusing on infertility (Becker) or IVF (Franklin).[31] A monograph by Bonaccorso (2009) also investigates the experience of people who underwent IVF in Milan, Italy. Like Franklin, she also provides excerpts from the narratives of people's experiences. Unlike Franklin, she does not make a political statement in opposition to IVF. She inquires about the views of gay couples as well as heterosexuals and couples without vested interest. Bonaccorso looks at IVF via gamete donation for an understanding of 'Italian kinship as a cultural form' (2009: xvi).

By providing narratives of donor women, Konrad (2005) shows that oocyte donation is a complex process whereby donors go through intensive treatment that is neither risk-free for their physical health, nor straightforward in emotional terms. She therefore argues that ova donation is tremendously different from sperm donation. For the surrogate mothers in the United States, who are paid for their 'service' (Ragone 1994), and for the ova donors in the United Kingdom, who are not paid (Konrad 2005), helping women to have children is a common rhetoric in their decision to donate.

Ethnographies of experiences with prenatal diagnostic procedures such as amniocentesis (Rapp 1999), ultrasound imagining (Mitchell and Georges 2000, Morgan 2000), and fetoscopy (Blizzard 2000) show that these treatments cause anxiety in women beyond the possible health risks for the women or babies. However, due to the excitement of 'seeing the baby' or 'knowing it is all right' the procedure is nevertheless pursued. 'Scientific knowledge' takes precedence over gestational embodied knowledge.

These few examples of ethnographies above concern women's experiences of assisted reproductive technologies. The motivation of the couples who pursue treatment, their physical and emotional states of being during treatments, disruptions that occur in their lives, the risks involved with the use of these technologies, and the governance of the female body are explored within the context of treatment narratives. Alternately, I rather focus on the experience of women before they start the treatment. I have included these examples to be able to locate my research in a larger picture of the ethnographies regarding IVF. My approach is to investigate infertility in various contexts from religious discourses to conflicts in extended families. My focus is on social relationships. I explore the ways in which social relationships influence childless lives, the attitudes towards procreation and assisted reproduction.

Theoretical attention to ART (more than infertility) emerged mostly in studies of kinship and technology in England and North America. Following the strong feminist objection to ART for being an invasive technology and a new means of male biopower on women's bodies in the 1980s (Arditti et al. 1984, Corea 1985, Crowe 1985, Franklin and McNeil 1998, Holmes et al. 1981, Klein 1989, Terry 1989), the 1990s saw a more balanced style of investigation of ARTs and infertility, as well as theoretically rich anthropological work.

Research in the domain of kinship since the advent of ART (although rising divorce rates and gay relationships are additional factors, as is rising academic interest in North America and Europe), due to a resurrection (Patterson 2005) or renaissance (Carsten 2004: 20, Clarke 2009: 2) in kinship, has been called 'new kinship studies' (Carsten 2004, Clarke 2008, 2009, Edwards and Salazar 2009, Patterson 2005, Strathern 2005). 'New kinship studies' scrutinize the ways in which ART lead to new ways of thinking about kinship (Strathern 1991b, 1992b, 1992c, 1994, 1995). Strathern (1992a, 1992b, 1992c) and Franklin (1988, 1997), following Schneider's (1968) analysis of American kinship, explored the ways in which kinship was reckoned biologically through the act of procreation (by blood or genes) in England. It was 'nature' which enabled procreation and which provided the 'facts of life'. These ethnographers drew attention to what happened to conceptions of kinship when faced with technologies that created kinship, and which shattered the entrenched assumptions about procreation and nature.[32] Franklin (1995) called the change in the perception of kinship and procreation a 'paradigm shift'. Nature seemed to need the helping hand of the 'enabling technology' (Strathern 1994). Science that was considered to bring 'miraculous reproduction' to 'desperate couples' could seem to provide new grounds for the facts of life (Franklin 1988, 1990, 1995, 1997).

Throughout the Middle East, there were no studies of this 'new kinship' until embryo and gamete donation as well as surrogacy became permitted practices in Lebanon (by religious authorities, Clarke 2006a, 2006b, 2007c, 2007d, 2008, 2009, Inhorn 2004, 2006b) and Iran (by civil authorities, Abbasi et al. 2008, Inhorn 2006b, Tremayne 2006). In Turkey (similarly to other Sunni Muslim countries), since third-party assisted reproduction is not allowed, the advent of IVF has not led to questioning the concept of kinship and the sources of knowledge for the facts of life. The law that bans third-party assisted reproduction aims to constrain practices that might threaten the 'sanctity of family' or the 'unity of the family'. Therefore the main focus of this research is not about the change in the perception of kinship in Turkey. The focus on kinship in this book lies on the social relationships among extended family members, which inform the experience of childlessness, rather than on the idea of biological relatedness and the recent changes in the definition of kinship.

About the Book

> Today we are discussing a very important topic that seems scientific, which is indeed scientific but which interests all of society, everyone, even the future of humanity as well as the academic circles: test-tube-babies. … This is a very important subject. It involves everyone. Some people are not directly related. Yet it concerns everyone in every aspect, whether it be ethical, religious, social or individual.[33]

The preceding words belong to the host of a weekly television debate programme with a wide viewership in Turkey. The host, Ali Kırca, strongly emphasizes the importance of *tüp bebek* (test-tube baby) for 'everyone' and 'humanity' in 'every aspect' in his introduction of the topic. The programme reflects the contested nature of IVF in the media and draws attention to the fact that there is 'a range of social, ethical and legal questions raised by new [reproductive] technologies' (Stanworth 1987: 2).

In approaching my research, I first sought to understand why people undergo IVF treatment. My initial question – which is the subject of the next (the first) chapter – was why they desired a child in the first place. Since, in many cases, a very fine line exists between desire and obligation, this inquiry at times turned into an exploration of why people feel obliged to have a child at all, a theme further elaborated on in later chapters. This question (why do people want children?) also challenges the 'naturalness' of the desire for a child.

The role of religion on the desire for IVF is the topic of the second chapter. I observed the prevalence of discourses on God's will in the narratives of childless lives in IVF clinics. Religion was also predominant in the daily lives of people I lived with during the second half of my research (in the two villages). These research experiences revealed the importance of scrutinizing how religious discourses and practices inform the experience of childlessness. The ways in which childless couples resort to religious rhetoric in order to constitute complete and normal gendered selves are also explored in this introduction.

The television discussion programme mentioned above featured a couple who had a child born with IVF. The programme host, Kırca, asked the couple if they reflected much before going for IVF. The response of the woman to the question was quite revealing:

> Yes, of course we thought it over. We were concerned about what others would say about it, what would the neighbours say, what would the relatives say. We considered its appropriateness by religion.

As is seen in the response above, the decision to opt for IVF involves checking its appropriateness with many sources. Religion is one of these.[34] It is also important that one's kin and friends find this decision appropriate. In addition to one's family, one's perceived social milieu directly influences the infertility experience.[35] Friends and acquaintances can be of support to childless couples for assisted conception treatments by providing them with names of IVF specialists or simply by encouraging them to get treatment. However, it is not uncommon for friends to be a source of pressure and suffering for childless couples. Childless people sometimes endure humiliation and ostracism, if not discrimination, brought on by prejudices and failure to meet social conventions. The third chapter explores the place of social relationships in the experience of infertility. Looking at the negotiations necessary to create complete adult identities and power in kin-neighbour social circles, I discuss the ways in which these negotiations impinge upon the 'quest for conception' (Inhorn 1994).

The next question Kırca asked the childless guests highlights another important field in this research:

> In Turkey people have certain presumptions about male infertility. Did you feel concerned about this; did you have unpleasant experiences when you decided to have IVF?

The husband of the woman who responded earlier replied that they did not have such worries and that they did not encounter any unfortunate incidents. The subtleties of the subject would make it difficult to say otherwise. The fourth chapter explores social relationships among men. The question posed above by Kırca reflects on the conflation of male infertility with sexual impotency. The chapter investigates the influence of manhood ideologies on men's and women's experiences of childlessness as well as on the decision to have IVF. Women may encounter social suffering due to infertility. Despite this, they very often take pains to shoulder the blame of infertility when their husbands have a fertility problem (Inhorn 1994, 1996, 2003b, 2004). I look for the possible reasons for such an endeavour by women.

Up to the fifth chapter, many of the possible reasons for conceiving a child *in vivo* (in a living organism, here in the female body) or *in vitro* (in glass, here via IVF) are discussed. In the fifth chapter the focus is on the demand for *in vitro* conception. The chapter investigates why people (women, especially) pursue endless cycles of IVF, and what kinds of insights this persistence in IVF treatment can give us about the lives and motives of the women who pursue them.

Another topic of inquiry in this book is the anthropological views on procreation. The gendered attitude to procreation and its influence on the decision to have IVF are key aspects of this study.

These are the key questions of this book. Yet they cannot be answered as if most women formed a homogenous category and as if ideas of parenthood were the same for everyone. For instance, social suffering due to childlessness is less common in the elite strata, such as the case in India described by Riessman (2000a, 2000b).[36] This is partly why working-class people who can hardly afford IVF were present in greater numbers in the IVF clinics (where I did research) than the more financially advantaged. The political economy of procreative decisions and attitudes is informed by a variety of factors. These factors, such as the nature of relationships in extended families, religion and hegemonic femininities and masculinities along with their subversions, are explored throughout the book.

It is also crucial to note that these factors not only indicate a variety of contexts, but also, perhaps more importantly, signify inequalities. A working-class woman who is in an IVF clinic may have overcome not only a financial challenge (which also marks inequality); she may also have a husband who is more influenced by manhood ideology, that complicates the decision to opt for IVF. She may also be living in an extended household under the authority of her mother-in-law, who objects to IVF. Her sisters-in-law may be making her feel incomplete and undesirable in the family because of childlessness. She may have no other route to a position of influence and respect without a child. These are only a few of the power inequalities she may want to overcome and need to negotiate in order to end up in an IVF clinic. They all indicate inequalities compared to the more elite, and compared to others in her social network who have children.

This book will underscore the explanations that figure prominently in the experience of childlessness (and in the decision to have or not to have IVF). I will identify repeated discourses, make explicit the influential ideologies, and uncover the relevant implications in the decision-making process for IVF. However, in the end, the book will reflect what I find most important, puzzling and prevalent regarding the experience of infertility and IVF in Turkey.

Notes

1. WHO 2004, DHS Reports 9.
2. The revised glossary is prepared by the WHO and The International Committee for Monitoring Assisted Reproductive Technology (ICMART). It is published in *Fertility and Sterility* 92:5, November 2009 and Human Reproduction 24:11: 1–5, 2009.
3. Lazi (*Laz*) are a minority living in the northeastern Black Sea region of Turkey. They speak Lazi (*Lazca*), as well as Turkish.
4. In fact, an important phase is deciding on an IVF specialist or IVF centre. This usually involves watching programmes and news about IVF on television, reading the relevant articles in newspapers, searching the web and listening to suggestions from friends and kin. Word of mouth is influential in such a decision. The cost of the treatment and the promotion of 'novel' procedures by different clinics also inform the final decision.
5. There were 122 IVF centres in twenty-two cities in Turkey, as of January 2010.

6. All the details about the legal practice of IVF and state funding in the book will reflect the conditions of the time when the research took place – despite the use of the present tense. This aims to give a relatively coherent picture of the research context and to prevent confusion.
7. Article 17 of the By-law for Centres for Assisted Reproduction published in the Official Gazette, 19.11.1996: http://www.mevzuat.adalet.gov.tr/html/20272.html.
8. For a thorough discussion regarding the number of embryos that can be transferred during IVF, please see Gürtin 2012b.
9. These three national social security institutions are *Bağ-Kur* (for employers, artists and tradesmen), *Emekli Sandığı* (for civil servants and military personnel) and *SSK* (for employees) which are attached to the Republic of Turkey Social Security Association (*SGK*).
10. See the website of the Prime Ministry for the pertinent legislation, as of 29 September 2008: http://rega.basbakanlik.gov.tr/eskiler/2008/09/20080929M1-1.htm.
11. For example in November 2006, news articles with titles such as '*Spermci Profesöre Hapis Cezası*' (Sperm-Swapping Professor Gets Prison Sentence) appeared in newspapers as well as on TV. A physician from a university hospital in Adana (The University of Çukurova) was found guilty of using his assistants' sperm to artificially inseminate women with infertile husbands. See for example, the article on http://www.milliyet.com.tr/2006/11/24/son/sontur26.asp dated 24 November 2006.
12. '*Sabah Sabah Seda Sayan*' (Seda Sayan in the Morning), appeared on weekday mornings on the TV channel *Kanal D*.
13. '*A'dan Z'ye*' (From A to Z), appeared at 3.15pm on weekdays, on the TV channel *ATV*.
14. '*Bebeğim*' (My Baby) appeared on a popular TV channel *ATV* from 21 December 2006 to 14 June 2007 every Thursday night. Despite the controversies it triggered, it never got high viewer ratings.
15. Another normalization practice is via religion. This is the subject of Chapter 2.
16. Polygyny is practised by some people despite its illegality in Turkey.
17. Not having a son is a strong drive for IVF for many reasons which will be discussed later in the book.
18. '*Meral Okyay'la Söyleşi*' [An Interview with Meral Okyay], was available at http://www.vatanim.com.tr/root.vatan?exec=cikolata_detay&hkat=1&hid=10477 on 23 March 2007.
19. See Gürtin (2009, 2010, 2011 and 2012a).
20. Gürtin (2009) also includes an overview of studies on the infertility experience of immigrants in Germany and the Netherlands. See for example Gacinski et al. (2002) for Germany and Van Rooij (2006, 2007) for the Netherlands.
21. Another pertinent argument Bonaccorso (2009: 11) makes is in regard to the problem of defining the Mediterranean as a 'cultural area

construct': a unified stereotypical presentation of the Mediterranean societies as pre-modern (Herzfeld 1987), marked by the honour and shame syndrome (Peristiany 1965, Pitt-Rivers 1965, 1977, Gilmore 1987). See also Herzfeld (1980, 1984), Llobera (1986) and Pina Cabral (1989) for critiques of a uniform Mediterranean cultural unit for anthropological analysis.

22. Scholars trained in Islam or a council of men with authority in the matters of Islamic law.
23. This will be discussed in Chapter 2.
24. The names of the people and places are pseudonyms.
25. See: Behar (1990, 1993), Behar and Gordon (1995), Bell (1988), Bertaux and Kohli (1984), Brody (1987), Bruner (1986), Crapanzano (1984), Cruikshank (1998), Frank (1979), Mishler (1986), Riessman (1987, 1988, 1993) and Robinson (1981).
26. The population of the coastal town was around 50,000 according to the 2000 census. Village Dere had 110 households whereas Village Tepe had 210 during my fieldwork.
27. Although Bosniaks are found in Turkey from the west to the east, most of them live in the northeast (Marmara region) of the county where Village Tepe is located.
28. The Koran is written in Arabic, so what I really refer to here is Arabic script. However, I want to emphasize that the intention was not to learn Arabic but only how to read the Koran.
29. Islamic attire here implies wearing a headscarf, as well as long-sleeved shirts and ankle-length skirts. Outside the home, it also involves wearing a long loose jacket. This was the dressing style of most of the village women.
30. See Fabian (1983) for a definition of the ethnographic present and his caution against denying the 'coevalness' of the ethnographer and the 'other' via using the ethnographic present, and a call by Sanjek (1991) for an 'ethnography of the present' or by Hastrup (1990) for the 'ethnographic present'.
31. It is important to note that these examples from ethnographic literature were published when IVF treatment was more physically demanding and time-consuming and less successful.
32. It is important to note that these views were expressed by these anthropologists around the time of the first UK legislation on assisted reproductive technologies (Human Fertilisation and Embryology Act) that took place in 1990. Thus, the debate should be evaluated with the time framework in mind.
33. The programme '*Siyaset Meydanı*' (Forum for Politics), on 26 April 2006, on the television channel *ATV*. This week's debate was on *in vitro* fertilization thanks to the second international conference titled 'Science and Moral Philosophy (Ethics) of Assisted Human Reproduction', which was held in Istanbul that week. One of the organizers of the

conference, Prof. Robert Edwards, the pioneer of IVF, was also present on the programme as well as other organizers. See Gürtin (2012a) for a discussion of this programme as well as the conference.

34. See Clarke (2007b, 2008 and 2009) for a discussion of moral propriety with regard to conception via IVF in Lebanon.
35. See Jenkins (2002) for an ethnography of childlessness in Costa Rica, which reveals the utmost pressure from friends and even from casual encounters to have a child. The voluntarily childless couple mentioned in the article feels compelled to have a child only to bring an end to incessant remarks about their childlessness.
36. Riessman (2000a, 2000b: 114–120) shows that in India, people of a higher socioeconomic class do not encounter stigma attached to infertility as much as women of lower economic classes.

Chapter 1

The Desire to Have a Child

This chapter lays out the reasons why people interviewed in this research – women in particular – desire children. In the first phase of the fieldwork that was undertaken in IVF clinics, conducting interviews with women pursuing IVF treatment, my initial question was always 'I am interested in your story from the moment you wanted a child to this moment. Could you please tell me first of all why you want a child?' I wanted to learn their stories, but knowing that my time was extremely limited, sometimes to only a few minutes, I wanted first to get the reasons for their decision to have a child.

It did not take long before I learned that there was no such decision. Mostly they simply wanted children and wanted to convince me that this was 'the natural way' of being an adult or a married person. In fact, most of the time my question was met with surprise: 'Who wouldn't want a kid? It is a natural thing' (*Çocuk kim istemez ki? Bu doğal birşey*). Beginning the interview with such a question proved to be a precarious method, for I was putting myself into the position of the impertinent researcher. In one sense, I was losing their trust from the beginning. As is widely known, building trust is vital to conducting in-depth interviews. In my case, it was especially important, as I was trying to elicit narratives on sensitive topics such as reproductive 'failure' and sexuality. I often needed a few more minutes before I could rebuild the trust I had lost at the outset of the interviews. Fortunately, in interviews that lasted longer than fifteen to twenty minutes, the negative effect of my first question vanished.

Despite its ramifications, I continued to begin my interviews with the question regarding the woman's reasons for desiring a child. This was mainly because I held the belief that it is not only words that are 'telling' (Wikan 2000). Surprise remarks, negations, silence and confusion are equally important responses. Thanks to this question, I could observe how bizarre the idea of not desiring a child seemed to people. I would argue that the strong responses of surprise and sharp criticism of the question reveal more about the conventions of adulthood than did the answers I could elicit during the rest of the interviews. The rhetoric of 'everyone wants a child', which is the usual first statement after the silence of surprise, indicates a compelling ideology of adulthood.

I received a wide range of reasons articulating women's desire for children, but responses generally emphasized a few themes. I have thus grouped the various reasons into two main categories. The first one deals with a metaphor frequently deployed in narratives for signifying a childless woman or a childless life: 'the tree that does not bear fruit'. In the course of analysing this metaphor, I point to the underlying reasons for a desire for children. The other category is boredom, or the joy that a child brings to life. In conclusion, it will be apparent that one can speak of an obligation to have children as much as a desire for them.

The Tree That Does Not Bear Fruit

'I hate this damned tree. I am going to cut it.' I am standing in front of a sour cherry tree with Selin in the garden in front of our house. We have been picking sour cherries all day in the strong sun. Wiping the sweat off her face with the back of her hand, she is talking to one of the sour cherry trees that has not been producing fruit in recent years. 'This is it. No cherries? That means I will cut you next year. I hate you. I will cut you.' Looking at her, I am having a hard time understanding what is taking place. I have never seen Selin use the word 'hate' so generously before. In fact, on reflection, I have never seen her hate anything or anyone. Gazing at her talking to the tree, which stands almost as a tribute to simplicity amidst eleven cherry trees adorned with blood-red fruits on dark green branches, all of this comes as a shock to me. She turns to me: 'Before cutting a fruitless tree, you should go to the tree and tell it that you will cut it. In fear of being cut, the tree gives fruit. If not, you cut it'.

She hates the fruitless cherry tree. This is the first time I have seen someone hate a tree, let alone affectionate Selin. How can someone hate a tree purely because there is no fruit on it? Now I see how people feel about trees that do not bear any fruit.

Two months earlier: in the South Clinic where I am doing research, I am sitting on a stool near the bed of a woman who is going to have an embryo transfer operation. She is lying on the bed. Hanife, who is now telling me about her life, has been married for twelve years. She tells me quite a lot about her suffering due to childlessness. She shows me her hair, all gone grey despite her young age (thirty-one). She says she is fed up with other people's disdain for her. This is her second IVF cycle:

> They tell you that no one wants to go near a fruitless tree. Does anyone go near a poplar tree? So they say you are similar to a poplar tree, as it has no fruit. So they say all kinds of things.

At home, late at night, I am going over my notes and writing in my diary before going to bed:

> Why the fuss about the fruitless tree from everyone? People inevitably go near fruitless trees: they go near them to have shade, to listen to the singing of birds. There are many beautiful fruitless trees in the world. If someone told me I was a fruitless tree, I would never take it as an insult. Besides I find poplars beautiful. What is she really talking about? What do they all really mean?

It took two months for me to realize what the fuss was about.

I was not yet ready to understand it, on my first day in the village, during the conversation I had with the very first villager I met. Her first question was if I was married. Her suggestion to me on hearing that I was single:

> Marry someone. Look at that tree. They will cut it one day. If you get married, you will have children. You will taste the world-fruit (*dünya meyvası*). What is a tree without fruit? Get married and have children.

I had to see Selin threaten a tree to understand how people detested fruitless trees. There was dislike, frustration and anger in Selin's demeanour towards the tree. Likewise, the childless women talked about experiencing dislike, frustration and anger. They were also implying that they were incomplete without fruit – or children. As a 'world-fruit', children were deeply desired in life. Who dislikes childless women? Why that frustration and anger? Why should they feel incomplete? Why the desire for a world-fruit? These are the questions I explore in this section.

I gradually gained awareness of the metaphor of the 'tree that does not bear fruit' (*meyva vermeyen ağaç*) or 'fruitless tree' (*meyvasız ağaç*) through the course of my fieldwork. Witnessing Selin threaten the sour cherry tree was a 'revelatory incident' (Fernandez 1986: xi) for me, as it helped reveal the links among emotions, interests, perceptions of childlessness and the desire for a child. These 'revelatory incidents' are the rewards of long-term participation in a culture, Fernandez asserts. He notes that these incidents are 'colloquial' since, first of all, 'they involve dialogue between members of a culture who differ from each other in generation or sex or class or occupation'. Moreover, they contain figurative expressions ('colloquialisms') and play with evocative tropes (Fernandez 1986: xi, xii). The play with tropes is apparent in this metaphor (childless women as fruitless trees), and the expressions of the metaphor I heard were often utterly evocative and figurative (nobody wants to go near a poplar tree).

I think it is important to understand this metaphor, for it emerged as an influential expression in the experience of infertility. It is frequently employed by people with children to denigrate childless women, as well as by childless women to explain their desire for a child. An overview of this metaphor will elucidate some of the reasons why people want – and why they are compelled to want – to produce offspring. It will also reveal some of the ways in which children and childless women are popularly conceived.

There are a number of ways to interpret a single metaphor (Basso 1976: 97). This will become apparent in going over the various interpretations of the metaphor by women. The way I am going to analyse these interpretations will be aligned with the ways in which they are perceived by women who use them. Thus the fruitless tree metaphor will reveal at least one assumption about childless women or childless marriages in each interpretation.

A Family Without Children is a Tree Without Fruit

– Why do you want to have children?
– Why, everyone wants to have a child. It is to have a fruit in marriage. (38 years old, married for 17 years, housewife, female-factor infertility)

- As they say, a family is better off with a child. As they say, a fruitless tree is disliked; there cannot be a family without children. (29 years old, married for 13 years, housewife, male-factor infertility)
- I really want to be a mother. A child is what makes a family. As there is no tree without a fruit, there is no family without a child. I cannot think of a family without a child; that will not be a family. Yet I do not want to leave my husband. I will never do such a thing. If IVF doesn't work, we will adopt a child. (21 years old, married for 4 years, housewife, male-factor infertility)

These are a few of the responses that use the metaphor of the fruitless tree (*meyvasız ağaç*) and the tree that does not bear any fruit (*meyva vermeyen ağaç*) to my question regarding the reasons for child desire. The responses above show how the ideology of the family requires children. A tree needs a fruit and a family (*aile*) needs a child (çocuk). A tree stands for a marriage or family and a fruit signifies a child in this context. This metaphor also informs the attitudes towards fruitless trees, or childless marriages. As trees that do not bear fruit are disliked, marriages without children are put in a precarious position. A family without children is inconceivable for people whose definitions of a family comprise children. This will become more apparent in further interpretations below.

A Child is the Fruit of Life/the World

- A child is the fruit of life. (32 years old, married for 12 years, housewife, unexplained infertility)
- I wish I had [a child], the world-fruit (if it is going to be good for us *hayırlıysa*).[1] (36 years old, married for 7 years, housewife, male-factor infertility)
- If there is a child, then there is a world-fruit at home. (42 years old, married for 26 years, housewife, female and male-factor infertility)

The tree metaphor is also used to signify life. The responses here belong to women, but a life without children can be quite inconceivable for men as well. A 'world-fruit' (*dünya meyvası*) implies the same. This world (also connoting 'life' here) is a place where one lives by virtue of being a parent. It is not uncommon for women and men to indicate that having a child is the meaning of life and that without children, they lose their reason to live. In Turkey, it is common 'to live for children' and 'to work for children': one works to 'give a good life' to her/his children. Childless people who work and earn well can be scorned for working in vain. Here follow a few more examples of the ways in which women conceive of and represent a child as the meaning and purpose of life:

- Your own child is different. When we have a child, we will live for her/him. Now we are living for nothing. If we have a child, our life will be meaningful. (22 years old, married for 4.5 years, housewife, female-factor infertility)
- A person strives for her/his child. We are striving in vain. What are you going to work for? For a child. Everything is meaningful when there is a child. (38 years old, married for 17 years, housewife, female-factor infertility)
- If we have a child, our future will have meaning, our life henceforth will have meaning. Meaning will come to our lives, we will not be living in vain. (35 years old, married 5 years, housewife, female and male-factor infertility)

A Woman without Children is Incomplete Like a Tree without Fruit

Incompleteness (*eksiklik*) is another concept implied by the image of the fruitless tree. Incomplete (childless) marriages/families and incomplete (childless) women are all signified by a fruitless tree – an incomplete tree. Women's desire for children is thus in order to have complete lives and identities. Below is a narrative about being an incomplete woman without children.

One day, in Village Tepe, we did not have the Koran class in the mosque but instead invited our Koran teacher (*hodja*) to Kibariye's house to join a discussion.[2] I had told Kibariye that I wanted to meet the whole class together so that I could pose questions to the women about family and children and learn their opinions. I hoped that women with children would talk more comfortably about infertility in the absence of childless women. However, contrary to my expectations, Kerime and another childless woman appeared for the discussion. Kibariye, aware that my research explored childlessness, had invited Kerime and Arzu. Kerime cancelled her plans to visit town in order to participate in our discussion. Sitting on the carpet around a low rectangular table with our Koran books on it, each of us (thirteen women and the *hodja*) read a couple of pages from the Koran. Our hodja listened to us and corrected our mistakes. After reading, I told everyone our main purpose for the gathering. So our discussion started, which continued partly in joy, partly in sorrow.

After the discussion, I chatted in another room with Ayla, who had her first child when she was nineteen, after three years of seeking a cure in every possible way including biomedical treatment and various folk practices. Our chat was interrupted by Kibariye, who approached us to tell me her 'real feelings and opinions' that she could not express near Kerime:

> Merve, I could not tell you inside, because I thought Kerime would be offended, but in my view, a child is the most important thing. There is nothing in the world more important than a child! There cannot be a life without a child. I could not say this near Kerime. She could be upset. But if you do not have a child, you are nothing! Your life, as well, is nothing! It is that important.

Kibariye indicated the central place of children in life and for women. But despite the measures Kibariye had taken, Kerime had already become upset by the discussion. At one point, while women were talking about what it means to be 'a woman', Kerime turned to Elif who was sitting next to her and whispered: 'How can I know about that [being a woman], I am not a whole woman, I am incomplete'.[3]

Kerime had whispered in such a low voice that it went unheard by the other women. Yet others had already mentioned incompleteness in reference to marriages: 'If you do not have a child in your marriage, you will definitely feel incompleteness (*eksiklik*)'. Kerime accepted herself as an incomplete woman. She shared the views of the others about this despite the pain it gave her. She was not questioning the dominant discourse or trying to change it; she perceived it as legitimate and reproduced it herself. This resembles Bourdieu's (1977) concept of symbolic violence. Her friends had garnered symbolic capital by having children. They could impose their opinions, which demarcated their superiority. This was not a deliberate form of coercion. On the contrary, they never intended to hurt Kerime, as is apparent in the measures Kibariye took in the discussion. Nevertheless, as a participant in the discussion, I had the chance to observe how women, including Kibariye, insisted on the incompleteness of a woman without a child, and to see how that distressed Kerime.[4]

I met Evcan at the North Clinic while she was resting after an embryo transfer operation. She was a 36-year-old high school graduate, who had been married for ten years, and worked as a salesperson. Her husband worked in a textile factory. They were living in Istanbul. They had tried artificial insemination four times before the IVF treatment. She hoped to conceive a daughter because, as she said – despite the fact that she had a job – she had been extremely bored during the last years. A daughter would be a friend to her. I asked her why she wanted to have a child. Her response reveals the incompleteness she felt (and was made to feel) in herself, her gender identity and in life:

> It is a huge incompleteness (*eksiklik*). I keep asking [myself] why I do not have a child. One feels incomplete. It is as if I am not a whole woman; I am something incomplete. Your family ostracizes you, society ostracizes you, and most especially, your husband ostracizes you. This is not something that can be explained. You are left all alone in the world. There cannot be a tree without fruit. You envy the ones with children. You say: 'Why don't I have a child?' That incompleteness is always there.

Having heard about the ostracism, when I asked her about her neighbours' attitude towards her childlessness, she told me that they were supportive, and brought the subject right back to not having a child:

> I am very bored when I am among other people, I feel incomplete. How can I explain this to you? It is as if you are a whole woman and I am a half woman. Being a half person: you cannot know that. Yet, I always tell myself, 'Let God give the *hayırlısı*. If it is not *hayırlısı*, I do not want it to happen.

Being infertile can engender incomplete gender identities in women. These women not only feel their family lives are incomplete, but also that their womanhood and adulthood are incomplete. As in Kerime's case, women want children in order to be accepted as adult women.

Inhorn (1996: 58–60) describes the incompleteness in the lives and identities of poor urban Egyptian women at three levels: infertility throws into question the very nature of a woman's humanity and sexual identity, as well as her gender identity. Infertile women's bodies 'are seen not quite as human' (1996: 58) because of the biological inability to produce a child. Infertile women are also seen as not quite female, having 'hidden male attributes' in the body. This research has not found incompleteness in these two levels: being human and being female as such. Incompleteness as lacking a full adult gender identity is, however, prevalent. For those people who endorse the view that the adult identity of a woman matures by virtue of bearing and rearing a child, a child makes a woman more of a 'woman' – in the eyes of others. Childless women never become full participants in the category of adult women by this reckoning.

Just like bearing fruit is in the nature of trees, bearing children is considered to be inherent in the nature of women. Women who cannot bear children fail their nature. It is also held to be natural (*doğal*), or in the nature of women (*kadının doğasında*) to want children. 'Every woman wants a child, it is natural', was a common first response to my question: 'Why do you want to have a child?' The parental desire that is represented as 'natural' reminds me of a booklet prepared by Organon, 'a research oriented pharmaceutical company' (Strathern 1992a: 57) in the United Kingdom. In that booklet, there is a reference to the naturalness of the desire for children. Strathern shows us that this discourse about nature – combined with a second instance in another booklet which presents the womb as natural – intends to stress how 'nature needs a helping hand' [the helping hand of technology]. In the Turkish discourse of parental desire or even of biological failing, the exact meaning of 'nature' (*Doğa, Tabiat*) is not clear unless, perhaps, it is women who are implied by nature. It is the nature of the woman that fails and needs a helping hand. When one resorts to IVF for assistance, the inability of 'nature' is not evoked as if it is in binary opposition to an 'enabling' technology (Strathern 1992a: 57).

Childless women express their distress because of their inability to do something that other women can do 'naturally', without effort, just like a tree blossoming and bearing fruit. Included in the definition of being a woman, or in the 'nature' of being a woman, is the expectation to produce offspring.

Childless women are thus stigmatized because of not meeting the standards of womanhood. Stigma, a concept introduced in the work of Erving Goffman (1963), emphasizes the discredited status of people who possess an attribute that does not meet social standards. The definition offered by Goffman (1963: 2, 3) is as follows:

> [A]n attribute that is deeply discrediting. Stigma can arise of [one] possessing an attribute that makes [that person] different from others in the category of persons for [that person] to be and of a less desirable kind – in the extreme, a person who is quite thoroughly bad, or dangerous or weak. [S/he] is thus reduced in our minds from a whole and usual person to a tainted, discounted one. Such

> an attribute is a stigma, especially when its discrediting effect is very extensive.

Goffman's (1963) work on stigma theory has been influential on Inhorn's (1996) work on infertility in Egypt and Riessman's (2000a, 2000b) work on infertility in Kerala, South India. The highlights of this definition that correspond to the experience of infertility, for Inhorn and Riessman, are that stigma is discrediting, makes a person less desirable and reduces a person from being whole and normal to being tainted and discounted. The same aspects of this definition apply to the experience of some Turkish women. I also find another aspect of stigma, discrimination against the so-called stigmatized, at least as important (Goffman 1963: 5). Childless women can be humiliated and ostracized. They are sometimes treated as 'undesirable wives' or more correctly, 'undesirable daughters-in-law'. Some of them are even made to feel that they are inferior to animals that can conceive.

Giving a Child/Son/Fruit

Giving and the ability to give are embodied in the expressions for producing a child. It is quite often the case that children are wanted in order to 'give children' (*çocuk vermek*) to one's husband (*koca, bey, eş*) and to 'give grandchildren' to parents-in-law (*kaynana* or *kayınvalide* for mother-in-law and *kaynata* or *kayınpeder* for father-in-law). Similar to the trees that are planted to give fruits (*meyva vermek*) to others, women give children. Thus, it comes as no surprise that women become distressed because of their inability to give to others:

> It makes me so sad, not being able to give a child to my husband. In fact, it finishes me. He is more enthusiastic than I am. If he becomes a father, worlds will belong to him.[5] I will give him the world if it [IVF] is successful. (28 years old, married for 7 years, housewife, female-factor infertility)

Giving a child appears as a deliberate action, in the 'rhetoric of the gift' (Layne 1999: 15), as well as part of a natural ability. Women naturally want to give children to their husbands and husbands' parents. However, it is worth underlining the fact that many women desire to give a child only because they see it as their duty. The ideology of giving is also marked in 'giving a son' to the husband and his family. Similar to the reasons for son preference described by Ilcan (1994b: 565), a son is desired because he will 'protect the family, pass on its traditions (such as its name and reputation), bring in the desired daughter-in-law, and inherit family property'. Although girls, by comparison, are seen as 'temporary members' of the household who will leave the family upon marriage, and perhaps for that reason are accorded less status (Ilcan 1994b: 565), most of the women I met in the clinics expressed their preference for a daughter.[6] A few women wanted to conceive a boy to please their in-laws.[7]

I met Saime at the South Clinic after an egg retrieval operation in her second IVF trial. She was twenty-three years old, had been married for four years, and had a daughter from her first IVF treatment. She was living in Istanbul but both her family and her husband's family were living in Sivas. She complained about the pressure she faced in their families' hometown to have more children. Saime was one of those women who are made to want children (a son in this case).

> I especially want a son because my in-laws want that very much. I already have a daughter; I would never initiate these [treatments] for a second child. My daughter would be enough for me. But I certainly have to give a son to these people. There is so much pressure. I started this treatment again due to their pressure for a son. Let's say, I go through all this, who knows if it is going to be male? Will I bear children until I have a male? Until when? 'Give a son!' 'Give a son!' I cannot! Anyhow, in our place of origin, whether you have a child or not, whether it is a son or not, it is always a subject of interest. But here [in Istanbul] nobody cares. The people of this place are civilized, first of all. Nobody knows anything about others. I am very comfortable here in that sense.

Women are made to desire a son, sometimes because of the pressure they face from their in-laws, and sometimes because it is the only way they can enjoy certain privileges. I do not only mean the well-known advantages of having a son, such as enjoying the esteemed status of being a mother-in-law one day. Sons are desired by women not only to secure their place in the patriarchy (White 1994: 36), to extend the patrilineage (1994: 57) or for the expected care in old age (1994: 63). Having a son may also have immediate desirable effects on a woman's life. Women can receive better treatment at home if they bear a son. Fadime's case is highly illustrative on this point (her husband also joined us later in the interview). Fadime had three daughters. She was living close to the eastern border of Turkey. She loved her daughters but she complained that her in-laws and the people in the village never considered them as children. Her husband told me he loved his daughters, but Fadime was quick to point out that he did not buy presents for his daughters, but for his nephews. She said that when they were alive, her in-laws pressured them to give them a grandson. I pointed to her that her parents-in-law had already passed away, yet she was having IVF treatment in pursuit of a son. She told me that she too wanted to have a son. Below are the various reasons she gave. Since the interview was an hour long and her reasons are scattered throughout the interview, I will only provide her statements directly related to this subject.

- They [friends and relatives] despise us. [They say] 'They have daughters, so what?' They do not see the daughters.
- When I was pregnant, my husband's brother's wife (*elti*) was also pregnant. She said, 'God will not give her any children [sons].' She treated me as if I was heartless (*hain*). That was how she was treating me.
- 'She cannot have a son, she is heartless.' They say, '[only] people who are not malevolent can have sons'. These [words] used to make me sad. I have gone through a lot.
- He [her husband] is dreaming of everything. 'I will do this, I will organize such a circumcision ceremony [for my son], I will have him circumcised as such…'
- They do not say she gave birth [about the women who give birth to girls]. But if it is a boy, for example, my husband's family says, 'she gave birth'. But if it is a girl, they do nothing [for the woman]. They do nothing. … They do not give food. Nothing. Milk, water, tea: nothing. But if it is a boy, ooooh, it is wonderful.
- If it is a boy, you are crowned.
- If it is a girl, they even take your money, and give back to you only a little of it. … Until his death, my father-in-law kept my husband's money; we were given a little pocket money.

Fadime's narrative illustrates the ways in which a woman is made to desire a child (a son in this case). She notes others' contemptuous attitudes towards her (including pejorative stereotypes), her husband's dreams of having a son, the unfair treatment (and ostracism) she received after delivering girls and even her own longing for the favourable treatment given to mothers of sons. She also mentions an economic disadvantage in having a girl. All of the above predicates the imposition of 'son desire' on women. In this instance, the rhetoric of the gift shows us how a child (or a son) becomes compelling.

In Turkey, where *ocak* literally means hearth but connotes household, family or family line, a son is required for the continuation of the *ocak* (Delaney 1991: 159) for some families. A man without sons, then, is considered *'ocağı sönmüş'* ('hearth is extinguished – his patriline has died out'). In one of the villages (Tepe), I was talking to women about having a son. An elderly woman pointed to a house and said: 'Look at that house. Its hearth is extinguished. There were three daughters in that house, no sons. The girls moved to other villages when they got married. The man and his wife died. There is nobody now in that house. If there were a son, then there would be a fire in the hearth (*ocağı tüterdi*)'. She was implying two different things. She meant that the house was empty because there was not anyone to live there, and that the patriline had died out. The women present expressed their sadness for that household.

It is not only women who see direct changes in their lives from having a son. Men can also see a change in their status at the moment they become fathers of sons. In Village Dere, when a son is born, his father goes to the village coffee shop (*kahve*) and distributes cake and buys tea for everyone there. All the men present in the *kahve* congratulate the man. When it is a girl, nothing is done. In Dere, Saadet and her husband – who were close friends with Elif's family – told us about the time they had their first daughter. They were able to have a daughter after sixteen years of a childless marriage. After the delivery of their first child, Saadet's husband went to the village *kahve*, and bought cake and tea for the men. He told me that everyone present was surprised at this behaviour and asked him why he was celebrating having a daughter. It was assumed there that anyone – unless they have a fertility problem – can produce a child, so only having a son is a special occasion to celebrate.

In Tepe, there are no such celebrations, and at first, people told me that there was no preference for sons in that village. However, after a while, I started to encounter people expressing a feeling of relief upon having a son. Since having a son is also an indication of virility, one of the women whose second child was a son told me: 'He [her husband] told me in relief, "At last I am normal, I am a male now in the eyes of others"'. She also told me that her parents-in-law were closer to their sons and daughters-in-law who had sons. The relationships between men and their parents were also affected by whether they had a son or not. However, in Tepe, not bearing a son was not a reason to pressure a son for divorce.

The Political Economy of Fruit on Trees

People plant fruit trees to make money from the sale of the fruit. Women, by this reasoning, need to bear children who will contribute to the family's financial power. The economic value of children is most apparent in villages. A family without children will not have the crucial manpower needed for farming, gardening, cattle breeding and so forth. For those who do not own their own land but work for others, an extra person means an additional contribution to the family budget via daily wages.

My friend Kerime, who was involuntarily childless (a temporary condition as she saw it), and I were walking by the tomato gardens in her village. We were walking from her house in the middle quarter of the village to the upper quarter, following an extremely steep path. Kerime walked trudgingly in contrast to my brisk stride because of the long-sleeved coat and headscarf she was wearing under the burning sun. While she stopped to catch her breath, we looked in admiration at the tomato gardens. The tomatoes were planted so neatly, unlike our (Elif and Selin's) tomato garden, which was much smaller and messy. Kerime told me that there were three thousand tomatoes in the garden we were looking at. Comparing it to the two hundred tomatoes in our own, I exclaimed: 'It must be loads of work!' Kerime sounded thoughtful when she responded: 'Merve, when you have children, does it matter if you have large fields or loads of work?'

In Kerime's village, there are no large farms, just fruit gardens. The main economic activity is cattle breeding. Since gardens and especially cattle bring in enough money to provide for a household, sons usually stay with their parents upon marriage. This is why sons are economically valuable. By contrast, women do not have economic value for their parents. They contribute to the economy of the families they marry into, by engaging in gardening and cattle-breeding activities. However, their most valued contribution comes indirectly, via 'giving children' (or sons/grandsons) to the family.

Children's economic value, therefore, impinges on the desirability of children. Children are desired more when they are considered as sources of economic benefit and wanted less when they are perceived as an economic burden. For urban people who pursue careers, for example, children are sources of expense with no anticipated economic benefit. This is one of the reasons for many couples to delay having a child for extended periods of time.

Trees That Do Not Bear Fruit Are Cut Down

A childless woman may be undesirable among her affines for not giving them a child. Another reason given for childless women's undesirability is that they may be found unattractive, unlikable (*sevimsiz*) – similar to a tree with no fruits. A sister of a childless woman in the village used the expression to describe her sister: 'She is *sevimsiz* like a fruitless tree, I pray for her to have a child'.

The following forms of the metaphor 'an infertile woman is a tree that does not bear any fruit' highlight the precarious position of women in their marriages:

- 'Nobody sits under a fruitless tree' (*Meyvasız ağacın altında kimse oturmaz*)
- 'Nobody goes under a fruitless tree' (*meyvasız ağacın dibine varılmaz*)
- 'A tree that does not bear fruit is stoned' (*meyva vermeyen ağacı taşlarlar*)[8]
- 'Fruitless trees are cut down' (*meyvasız ağacı keserler*)
- 'Nobody wants a tree that does not bear fruit' (*meyva vermeyen ağacı kimse istemez*)

Sometimes childless women's female in-laws or friends use these metaphors to remind them about their undesirability. They are also used as a threat to women (just like Selin threatening the sour cherry tree) for not giving a child. A mother-in-law who wants her son to divorce may employ one of these expressions to her daughter-in-law to point to the possibility of a divorce.

These expressions emphasize the ebbing interest of men in their wives. The sister of the childless woman mentioned above said: 'Why should her husband go home after work? She is *sevimsiz*. There is no fruit of joy at home'. A man, according to her, loses interest in his childless wife or dull home (*yuva*) that lacks children, and spends more time outside.

The metaphor of the fruitless tree, therefore, also speaks of the ambiguity regarding the future of the marriage as well as the diminishing affection between the conjugal spouses. The expressions above are not only linguistic tools, but metaphorical concepts (Lakoff and Johnson 1980: 6–9) that reveal how childless women are conceptualized via the use of 'everyday experiences'. The reason why I faced difficulties in understanding this metaphor was that fruitless trees are not part of my own everyday experience. Between the metaphorical concepts are relationships of entailment (1980: 6–9). 'Fruitless trees are cut down' for example, implies that childless women are undesirable, which in turn implies that they are not needed anymore, i.e. they are useless. In other words, cutting down trees, not wanting fruitless trees, are expressions – 'metaphorical entailments' – that refer to the undesirability and so to the uselessness of childless women.

This reckoning sheds some light on the dynamics of the perception of infertility, as well as on the understanding of the maltreatment that childless women sometimes encounter. I do not intend to imply – as Lakoff and Johnson (1980) do – that it is always by metaphors that conceptualization is done. But when metaphors are used, they point to the ways in which 'analogies are drawn between things, in the way certain thoughts are used to think others' (Strathern 1992a: 33). To understand culture in that sense, therefore, it is worthwhile – but not sufficient – to look at 'how trope itself can operate as an organising principle' (Wagner 1986: x).

Having said this, I want to point to the risk involved in the over-emphasis of the metaphor as such. Bearing in mind the above analysis of the fruitless tree metaphor, it is possible to argue that undesirable qualities such as uselessness are attributed to the childless woman. Observation can reveal the emotions that go with this metaphor: anger, frustration and desire to get rid of the tree (the woman). Stereotypes such as incompleteness and uselessness become explicit with the metaphor. An analysis of the fruitless tree metaphor thus provides an invaluable insight into the conceptual significance of motherhood. Since these are crucial for an understanding of the experience of infertility and so of the demand for IVF, I started with an analysis of this metaphor.

Yet one cannot tell, only by looking at the metaphor, why people want children, what they experience when they do not have a child, and why they decide to get IVF treatment. It will be apparent in the next half of the chapter that this metaphor is not sufficient for explaining all the perceptions, attitudes, motives and experiences related to child desire. The remaining part of the book will show that it is also far from delineating a full picture of people's perceptions of procreation, infertility and gender ideologies.

Delaney (1991), who did ethnographic research in a village in central Turkey from 1980–1982, asserts the predominance of the use of the metaphor 'the seed and the soil' in Turkey.[9] She explains this metaphor by drawing on a 'monogenetic' procreation narrative in which the field (woman) is sown (impregnated) with the seed (sperm/man). To this end, she associates this procreation story with a range of issues such as gender, kinship, cosmology, religion, honour and shame. The importance attributed to having a son and to endogamy, for example, reflects the importance given to the creative power of men (1991: 36, 76). Claiming that man, in Turkish reckoning, is metaphorically analogous to God in his creative role (in impregnating the seed), and that there is an alliance between God and men, is the ground of her theory of procreation (and so of gender). According to this theory, the alleged alliance with God legitimates and perpetuates the powerful position of men. It therefore explains the conditions that generate patriarchy (1991: 34–35).

Delaney's analysis of procreation in Turkey has contributed to anthropological theories of procreation and gender in various ways. The most important contribution she makes is her explicit attention to European perceptions of procreation rather than focusing on the exotic other. In *The Seed and the Soil* (1991), she aims to understand Western perceptions of procreation, and challenge the assumptions that they alone are 'facts', while the procreation theories of others are 'cultural'.[10]

Delaney (1991) puts emphasis on the relation between procreation and gender rather than the common anthropological practice – after Malinowski (1929) – of looking at the relation between procreation and kinship. She criticizes the Western anthropological practice of turning to the knowledge about procreation in order to understand kinship (1991: 9). Anthropologists writing in the area of assisted reproductive technologies have indeed continued the tradition of relating procreation to kinship, making contributions to the anthropology of kinship in the form of 'new kinship studies'. However, I find Delaney's emphasis on gender rather than kinship a useful vantage point for understanding the implications of childlessness, the topic of this research. The perception of infertility and the ways in which it is lived and expressed are contingent upon feminine and masculine ideologies. A focus on gendered procreation is particularly useful for the main argument of this book.

Delaney's ethnographic study of Turkey thus has obvious contributions to anthropological theory and to ethnographic studies in Turkey. On the other hand, her use of the metaphor 'the seed and the soil' in building a cosmological universe along with a theory of procreation may be taken as an example of the over-interpretation of metaphors.[11]

Neyzi (1994: 213), in a review of *The Seed and the Soil*, finds Delaney's procreation theory surprisingly coherent.[12] This coherence is because her depiction of cosmology rests entirely on one metaphor (seed and soil). Delaney may have fallen into the trap of taking too seriously 'the most gifted or knowledgeable philosopher' one finds (Keesing 1985: 202). Keesing's concerns on the topic bear due consideration: 'Have we invented cosmologies, theologies, beliefs constructed out of other peoples' metaphors?' (Keesing 1985: 202). Keesing identifies the use of 'the most gifted or knowledgeable folk philosopher' as problematic in the analysis of metaphors. He cautions against turning the personal views of such informants into elaborate theories of which other locals are unaware. 'Attempting to uncover the native theory of procreation or the person means ignoring the multivaried nature of cultural discourses' (Busby 2000: 86). As Beller-Hann (1999: 115) highlights, Delaney gets the most crucial statement upon which she grounds her procreation theory from a quote from Meeker (1970: 157):[13] 'If you plant wheat, you get wheat. If you plant barley, you get barley' (Delaney 1986: 497, 1991: 33). We therefore cannot be sure if she has also been taken in by a 'knowledgeable or gifted' informant or if she has sacrificed the variety in discourses and practices in favour of constructing a uniform grand theory.

Essentialization of data for a coherent meaning and a consistent theory by means of a metaphor can also be evaluated within the framework of symbolic anthropology. Geertz, who was a pioneer of symbolic or interpretive anthropology, was also criticized for failing to include the people's voices that led to his interpretations (Connor 1984: 271, Shankman 1984: 269, Varisco 2005), for generalizing without sufficient evidence from the field, such as making claims for 'the Balinese' when it was only Java where he undertook his research (Hobart 1999: 117) for generalizing and centralizing one local and perhaps peripheral meaning of the 'trance' (*nadi*) to the Balinese, for forsaking other more relevant meanings (Connor 1984: 274), as well as for essentializing through symbols (Obadia 2007), and for essentializing religion (Asad 1993: 29–33, Limberis 2000: 374) and Islam (Varisco 2005).[14]

I find Delaney's (1986, 1991) analysis of the seed and soil metaphor an example of the way Geertzian anthropologists look at symbols to see how they 'shape the ways social actors see, feel and think about the world' (Ortner 1984: 129). This should indicate that I am not after endless contextualization, but rather after a more explicit relationship between contexts informed by people's engagements and disengagements with them.

Joy, Occupation

> *Once upon a time there was a very rich man, who had everything but joy in life. He had a poor neighbour with a joyful family. One day, the rich man told his neighbour: 'How joyful you are!' His poor neighbour responded: 'I have a golden ball'. He was implying that he had children, but the rich man did not understand this. He bought a golden ball – because he was a rich man – and brought it home. So, he placed the golden ball in his house, and waited, but nothing happened. Then he said to the poor neighbour, 'I, too, bought a golden ball'. The poor man explained: 'I have children'.*

> What can you do [at home with your husband] as time passes by? A monotonous life begins. Then what happens? You want a change; you want a baby ... Only two people, that is different.[15]

Sitting on a stool next to her bed, I was listening to Yaprak, who had just had an embryo transfer. Despite the fact that she worked (as the human resources manager of a private firm) during the day, she narrated this golden ball story in order to elaborate on the inevitability of boredom in a childless marriage. She was a 28-year-old woman living in Istanbul, married for seven years. She is one of many people who have emphasized the need for a child in marriage in order to escape boredom. The same golden ball story was also recounted by a friend in Village Dere. She married the only son of one of our neighbours when I was in the village. When I asked her why she wanted to have a child, she explained that the main reason for having a child lies in the story of the golden ball, that is, children are the joy of a marriage.

I was often bewildered when the desire for a child was articulated with a reference to avoiding boredom. Having joy (*neşe*) in marriage and a pastime (*meşgale, meşguliyet*: something that keeps one busy) in daily life come to the fore among reasons for child desire. Without a child, life is regarded as monotonous and 'empty'. As a single and childless woman I also frequently encountered such comments: 'Get married and have children. A life without children is insipid'.

When caring for children is the preoccupation of women, a childless life means a life with nothing to do other than housework (Inhorn 1996 on Egypt). Children are taken to be the riches (Thiessen 1999), the pleasure of life (Delaney 1991) and a life without them is assumed to be 'uninteresting and lonely' (Handwerker 1995 on the Han in China).

Here are a few of the many examples (from interviews in the IVF clinics) in which 'joy of life' and boredom sharply indicated the desire for a child:

- Let there be a child at home. We will play [with her/him], spend time. Our dream is having a child wandering around at home. (33 years old, married for 6 years, housewife, female-factor infertility)
- There is emptiness [inside the house] ... I am bored at home myself. If I had a child, I would not be bored at home. I am bored all alone. (23 years old, married for 2 years, housewife, female-factor infertility)
- A child is the joy of a house, is the foundation of a marriage. Being a parent is a very different feeling. I want to feel that, what can I say? (28 years old, married for 7 years, housewife, female-factor infertility)

Nisa is a forty-year-old woman married for seventeen years. She lives in the southeastern part of Turkey with her husband. I met her at the North Clinic when she was waiting for her egg retrieval operation.

> As it is with any other mother and father, it [our desire to have a child] is natural. It is our only wish. May God not let a tree stay fruitless and a person without a child. We had operations twice; nothing came of them. We tried IVF. This is the third time. *İnşallah* [hopefully, God willing] it will be all right. Inside four walls, it is very difficult. Time does not pass. The house is very empty. I try to avoid distress by immersing myself in watching television. The problem belongs to my husband ... If I have a child, I want to rear her/him, take care of her/him, go shopping for her/him, dress her/him.[16] Like this, it is all looking at each other's faces. In the evenings, we watch television, drink tea but nothing else. But I wish we had a child so that we could be occupied with her/him. We want children for the same reason young people want children. It is our most natural right like it is for others. Everyone has children, you look at them and want one for yourself, you say, 'I wish I could have one, too.'

> Of course everything is in God's will. One never stops hoping for a child from God.

Nisa's story is adorned with themes that prevail in other narratives: monotony in the marriage, the child as a source of entertainment for the couple and occupation for the mother, the impact on the couple of seeing other people with children and the analogy of a fruitless tree. Desiring children is seen as 'the most natural right', and it is assumed that everyone wants a child, because it is regarded as 'natural'. These themes recur in most of the narratives elicited from childless women in the hospitals. I will go into the other common themes later but here it seems worthwhile to note that many of these women are housewives who do not have much to do in their daily lives other than domestic chores and watching television. Children, therefore, become the primary means of occupation and entertainment for women during the day. Moreover, without children it is held that nothing is shared between husband and wife. When the husband comes home after work, there is nothing to do together but watch television. Nonetheless, even those women who undertake economically productive work can have the same complaints about their marriages, as in the case of Yaprak. Boredom and emptiness seem to be embodied in a childless life.

Since boredom and emptiness appear as entrenched markers of child desire, I want to elaborate on their meanings. Boredom is an 'underresearched topic' in social anthropology (Musharbash 2007: 307). It is more widely studied in philosophy and sociology, especially along the axis of universal-timeless (Kuhn 1976) and historical (Goodstein 2005, Svendson 2005) phenomena. It is now widely assumed that boredom is a Western phenomenon that should be located in modernity. Svendson (2005: 153), who has written about boredom through the framework of philosophy, sees it as a major problem brought by modernity. He emphasizes the implications of the lack of tradition on people's lives in modernity: 'When traditional structures of meaning disappear', meaning has to be sought individually, and the failure to find a meaning eventually engenders boredom. In Svendson's analysis, therefore, boredom is not only historically situated but is also associated with the lack of meaning in life. This is also reflected in Spacks (1995), who sees boredom as 'a common signifier of ethical crisis' in modernity, and Goodstein (2005) who depicts boredom as a 'malaise of modernity' as well as an 'experience without qualities'.

Attributing boredom to modernity and to the West fails to acknowledge the appearance of boredom in many other contexts. I hold that boredom is not always a consequence of alienation or the diminishing role of religion in people's lives, both of which are usually regarded as consequences of modernity. To understand boredom, one should look at people's quotidian experiences. In the case of this research, for those people who are practising devout Muslims, childlessness still appears as a crucial marker of boredom. Therefore, I do not find that boredom in the narratives of childless women (in my research) is a by-product of modernity.

Boredom, in the narratives of Turkish women I have interviewed and observed, reflects more of an emotional state of disturbance or suffering that derives from the inability to reach a certain lifestyle, a life goal, a means to enhance one's (gender, adult) identity. The lifestyle or life goal that is sought after is not a product of modernity (although the means to achieve this goal may certainly be): motherhood and the concept of a family with children do not belong to modernity as such.

The first two definitions of boredom (*sıkıntı*) in the dictionary of the Turkish Language Association (*Türk Dil Kurumu*) online appear as follows:

1. Psychological fatigue, suffering, torment due to having nothing to do, monotony, weariness etc.
2. Perennial fatigue, suffering due to a problem, disorder.[17]

Fatigue is a distinctive aspect of boredom in the dictionary. It refers to emotions or a psychological state. The presumption is that one gets mentally and emotionally tired when there is nothing interesting to do, as opposed to the physical body that gets tired due to excessive physical exertion. Monotony and weariness, sometimes synonymous with boredom, are also included in the definition.

Another marker of boredom is 'suffering'. This meaning, in my view, is particularly salient to what the childless women mean by boredom. It explains why women would want to end this emotional state: they do not want to stay unhappy or to suffer.

'Having nothing to do', which is implied in the dictionary as a reason for boredom, also appeals to the narratives of childless women. It is how they articulate their need for a child at home/in marriage/in life. A child will provide the busy pursuits they look for in life. It is not that childless people do not have anything to do in life. It is rather that they do not have the thing they look for in life. It is true that they complain of vacuity in their lives, but this is because they tend to put children in the centre of their lives, and in the absence of children, the centre of their lives becomes a huge void. They would not want to replace children with anything else because they would not be able to conceive of a possible substitute in the first place.

This was much the same in the two villages. On one occasion, I was chatting with Firdevs, a young woman with whom I had the chance to make very good friends in Village Dere. She is twenty-seven years old and lives with her parents, her brother and her sister-in-law. Her two other brothers and their families live a few metres away. Firdevs' family is originally from the eastern Black Sea region, as is apparent in their dialect and customs. Firdevs is a big help to her parents in the garden. She works from early morning to evening as she plants, weeds, picks fruit, makes molasses, transfers forage from fields to the garden and so forth.

After Firdevs finished junior high school, she took Koran classes for two years. She wanted to continue school or start working, but her father was opposed to both. Her father never allows her to leave the house without her mother or brothers. He rigorously monitors his daughter's contact with the outside world. Nonetheless, she is free to enjoy her time at home and in the gardens however she likes. Her life, thus, is composed of her parents, gardens, domestic housework, needlework, and inevitably, of religion.

It was the month of holy Ramadan. I was at her home to participate in the fast-breaking dinner in the evening. After a tiring day of making molasses, we went home to chat. As I did often in my conversations with women, I started to talk about marriage and children. I asked her opinion on getting married. She was already well above the standard age of marriage in the village. She looked at me and said: 'So, what shall I do if I do not get married? I am not going to school; I am not working. When there is a child, I can be occupied (*oyalanırım*) with that'.[18]

Here I want to reflect on my feelings on this exchange with Firdevs. When Firdevs said she foresaw having a child as her only major occupation in the future, I found myself comparing her life up to that point with my own. Firdevs' social circle was small, and mostly composed of relatives. She had never encountered any academic challenges such as entrance exams for university. She did not have to take endless additional courses to succeed in exams, nor did she even have to worry about them. She had never experienced the difficulties of making friends, managing friendships, coping with misunderstandings and unfair treatments. In such absence of socialization, she never had to be concerned about constituting and representing her identity. She had never gone through any sort of experience related to having a love life. She had never had her heart broken. She was sad not to have a job, but this also meant she had never faced the challenge of applying for a job and succeeding in it. Throughout her life, she has had the gardens and her family, and plenty of time to think about marriage and children. When she gets married, her only occupation will be domestic chores and her only worries will be – if she has any – managing her relationships with her in-laws as well as having a child. If she is not able to have a child, it will be the first major frustration that she experiences in life. That may also bring her other kinds of problems that she would not have experienced up to that point, such as challenges in her social relationships. In addition, her life will be devoid of goals, responsibilities, joy and entertainment.

The women in the villages work in the gardens in spring and summer. However, during fall and winter there is nothing much to do in the gardens. They complete their housework in the morning and then take a nap, watch television, do needlework or visit each other, where they again watch television or do needlework. The ones who do not have gardens or who start living in an apartment in town after marriage have much less to do throughout the year.

It is usually the first few years of a child's life that are invoked when the child is seen as a source of joy and an enjoyable pastime. The typical image is of a baby or toddler. Envisioning the first lovely years of bringing up a child, childless women delineate the sort of entertainment that they long for. The later stages of childhood are not found in women's narratives. However, my interviews with two voluntarily childless women, a bank manager and a physician, reveal that these women considered children's further development when they decided against having a child. For them, it seems difficult to bring up a child after the first years: there are too many outside threats, such as the increase in drug use and the enormous expenses involved in rearing a child. These women are wealthier than most of the women I interviewed in the clinics, but they seem to have calculated every financial as well as emotional aspect of having a child.[19]

Freedom of Mobility

Kerime, from Tepe, has been married for thirteen years. In my last visit to her house, I asked her about the major problems she faces due to being childless. She told me that just like any other man, her husband wanted to be a father. Although he never pressures her, she feels sad about 'not being able to make him a father' (*onu baba yapamamak*). The second problem she mentioned was:

> For example, I do not like to go out of our quarter alone. However, if I had a child, I could take her/him with me and go out.

For Kerime, having children will add to her freedom of movement, just as it will enable her to become a full member of the female community and enjoy taking care of children as other women do. Freedom of movement was more explicitly expressed by the mother-in-law of a young woman, Meryem, who got married the summer I was in Dere. Meryem is seventeen years old. Her parents' house is on the way to town from our house. Her family comes from the eastern Black Sea region of Turkey. I used to visit them each time I walked down to town, which enabled me to set up a good relationship with Meryem and her mother. Two months after her marriage, her mother took me to Meryem's new house, under an hour away.

Meryem lives in an apartment in a three-storey building. Her house is close to the highway and far from the village centre, which makes it difficult to enjoy village life. While we were having tea on the balcony, Meryem's mother-in-law arrived. Meryem is not submissive towards her mother-in-law. On the contrary, she is extremely outspoken.

Meryem does not have many daily activities. By noon, she is finished with all her chores. After that, she usually goes to sleep, watches television or does needlework. Her mother-in-law joked about her laziness. 'Meryem, you are lazy. You cannot even do that needlework. ... She is always sleeping.' Meryem never goes out of the house because her husband does not allow her to do so. Her mother-in-law told her that she would enjoy more freedom when she had a child:

> Her husband [she is talking about her son] is very jealous. But don't worry, my daughter, mine was the same in the beginning. Then, when there is a baby, they start to change. Your husband will change, too.

On the way to Meryem's house, I had asked Meryem's mother if her daughter visited her when she came to the weekly bazaar nearby. Her response reveals a similar association of having children with increased freedom:

> Of course she comes to the bazaar but she comes with her husband. Her husband is very jealous, he does not send her to the market, he does not let her do anything. Men are like this initially but after a couple of years, especially when there is a child, they never care about it. At that time, a relaxed period for women starts, and then it goes on like that. When there is a child, men leave their wives totally free.

Both for Kerime who was thirty-seven and Meryem who was seventeen, a child meant increased freedom of mobility and less boredom. Kerime was a very outgoing woman who enjoyed making house visits. It would be much easier for her to go around with a child. For Meryem, life was dull, with nothing to do. She could at least visit her mother's house if she had a child.

The Right to Have a Child

Answers obscure as much as they reveal. This includes the answers to the question at the heart of this chapter: Why do you want children? I started the chapter discussing the surprise that this question engenders in people. Asking people why they want to have children presumes that it is children they are after. In an IVF clinic, where people come for help conceiving or 'to produce children', one may assume so. Yet this assumption may be misleading, and so may my question be.

One could also ask a similar question in different words: Why do you want to be a parent? Insofar as people visit IVF clinics in order to be parents (Thompson 2005), it makes sense to inquire about their expectations of motherhood and fatherhood. As Inhorn notes for urban poor Egyptian women: 'It is not only children that are deemed missing from infertile women's lives. It is motherhood itself – with all that it entails for a woman's existence and her gendered identity' (1996: 64–65, 2000). Indeed, the symbolism of the fruitless tree and the stereotypes it entailed served as powerful incentives for motherhood.

Having said this, it is not only 'desire' for children or parenthood that makes people pursue endless assisted-conception treatments. This brings us to another point that the question conceals. Motherhood is essential for attaining one's adult gender identity, for establishing good relations within one's extended family, for ensuring marital stability, for enjoying participation in the adult world and so forth. When there is a period of involuntary childlessness, motherhood becomes even more compelling as a way to end the concomitant emotional and social suffering. As will be shown throughout this book, the line demarcating desire from obligation is not always straightforward.

Another crucial aspect of this question is that it may lead to misunderstanding, particularly when it is asked of IVF patients. This question elicited feelings of unfair treatment among a few IVF patients, or even feelings of discrimination. They interpreted the question as disputing their right to have a child by attributing to them an importunate desire. At these times, they would insist that they had at least as much right as other people to have a child and that this was natural. I concede their point, for I am aware of the likely implications of such a question. IVF patients interpreted the question as discriminating against them because they had already been accused of being selfish for pursuing IVF instead of adopting a child. Sandeloswki's (1993: 39) remark about American couples reinforces this point:

> The desire of infertile couples for what most other couples want, expect, and get is called into question and interpreted as racist, eugenic, and selfish. Moreover, the desire of a couple to bear their own child or to adopt a child who could have been their own is deemed irrational, obsessive, and suspect only in infertile couples. Normally fertile couples who desire children neither forego, nor are they expected to forego, having their own children in the interests of adopting children already born and without parents. Importantly, infertile couples are asked to be 'more virtuous, more selfless [and] more liberated' than the vast majority of fertile couples (Lasker and Borg 1987: 190), and better to handle the constraints against which all human beings make choices.

Apparently, childless couples who pursued IVF did not like anyone to question their right to have a child. For most of them, having a life without a child was not natural, just as a tree without fruits.

Being a parent, and devoting a life to one's child was what described adulthood and so it was hard to visualize their future as an adult without being a parent. Parenting appeared as the main responsibility one takes on as an adult, and the major occupation without which life is empty and meaningless.

The Motherhood Rhetoric

'To fully understand the consequences of infertility and its relationship to high fertility, the notion of pronatalism – beliefs about the importance of motherhood, fatherhood, and the desirability of having children – must be interrogated' (Inhorn 2003a: 7). This motivation to understand the reasons for one's desire to have a child is the vantage point for understanding infertility as well as fertility for many ethnographic studies that reveal that motherhood is what creates womanhood, one's full adult identity or even in some cases, one's 'human' identity (Inhorn 1996: 58). As mentioned before, an enquiry into the desire for a child has also been the vantage point for this research.

During the period of my research, discourses on motherhood were also reproduced in television serials with high viewing levels – and they still are. 'To be able to make sacrifices for one's child' as a marker of motherhood was a dominant script in these serials. In one of them, *Binbir Gece* ('1001 Nights'), the female lead had sex with her boss for money in order to fund her son's bone marrow transplant. The serial was covered extensively in the media. The praise for her motherhood greatly superseded the critiques of her morality for engaging in a sexual relationship for money. Views of celebrities who defended the woman's act established motherhood as a sacred role capable of sacrifice (*fedakarlık*). Such discourses reify motherhood to the extent that mothers are seen as the only people who can understand, feel and do certain highly regarded things, while others cannot.

The motherhood rhetoric is also constantly perpetuated by the state. As Navaro-Yashin (2002: 2–6) suggests, the state cannot be limited to the public discourses of a governing institution; it is found in many disguises – 'faces of the state' – everywhere in public life. With regards to the ideology of motherhood, the faces of the state are even more disguised, when motherhood is taken as a natural need/drive/essential aspect/right of womanhood.

Sending troops to fight in a foreign land and the large number of deaths due to the war with the terrorist group PKK (Kurdistan Workers' Party) are often reprimanded with the powerful discourse 'let not the hearts of mothers burn' (*anaların yüreği yanmasın*).[20] Yaraman (1999: 121–124) points to the political campaigns in Turkey that promise childcare facilities, maternity leave and payment of childcare costs for working women. These political promises equate women with mothers. According to Arat (2000) and Sirman (1989), this gender ideology was already present in the first years of the Turkish Republic (1920s and 30s). However, Gümüşoğlu (1996) reveals that the motherhood rhetoric has gained ground over the years. Gümüşoğlu looks at all the textbooks (925 books) of the primary and high schools from the first day of the Republic to the 1990s. After 1950, the image of the Turkish woman turns into a housewife and a mother, busy with domestic work such as cleaning, cooking or taking care of children. Similarly, Saktanber (1993: 216–217) analyses Turkish radio programs targeted at women (between 1939 and 1980). The predominant images of women in these programs are 'a wife and a mother in the context of the family' and 'a human being in the world, a citizen in society'. Childcare, health and familial relations are the most popular subjects in these radio programmes targeted at women.

Rising Islamism in Turkey also promotes motherhood as a primary role for women. Acar's (1993, 1995) research on female Islamist university students shows that the majority of the girls she interviewed were going to university not to get a job but to become educated mothers in the future who can bring up children well. Turkish Prime Minister Erdoğan's promotion of motherhood was explicit in his speech to mark International Women's Day in 2008.[21] He suggested that Turkish women bear at least three children so that Turkey does not face the threat of an ageing population in the near future. He repeated this advice on several occasions after that date and warned against the dissolution of the institution of the family: 'If the institution of the family dissolves, it means our nation is facing a collapse. So, I insist on the family'.[22] This is despite the low availability of childcare facilities. Only 4 per cent of working women with a child under six years old take their children to a day nursery in Turkey. Usually it is mothers of the husbands (21 per cent), women's own mothers (9 per cent), or their elder daughters (10 per cent) who care for children (KSGM, 2003 figures). When they do not have such support, women have to quit work. The difficulties inherent for working mothers in Turkey are also reflected in the fact that at least half of the women in academia are single (Acar 1993: 74), according to the findings of a study by Acar (1991).

Erdoğan's message for Women's Day is important not only for its conflation of womanhood with motherhood, or the predominance of motherhood as a state ideology, or the governance of women's bodies by the state via intervening in women's reproductive choices. It also highlights the family as a crucial ideological keystone that is perpetuated and governed by the state. Erdoğan's words above reveal the extent to which the hegemony of the family with children reigns in the discursive practices of the state.

The reasons for the desire to have a child have been a popular subject of enquiry in various studies that argue that conceiving a child is a common expectation of a woman as well as of an ideal marriage.[23] Similarly to what I have underlined about the use of the motherhood mandate in Turkey by the media and the state, in these studies, the 'ideology of the motherhood' (Gupta 2000) assumes a conflation of womanhood with motherhood. Widge (2002), speaking on the Indian context, comments that fertility defines womanhood. Among the Han in China, (Handwerker 1995: 365) one of the reasons given for the desire for a child is: 'If I don't have the ability to give birth, I am not a woman'. The second and the third chapters of this book will make explicit the ways in which a childless woman can be made to feel incomplete as a woman.

A strong motivator for being a mother is to form stable and peaceful conjugal bonds with the presence of children. Although polygyny is illegal in Turkey, in Vietnam and in India, it may still be practised, especially in rural populations when a woman cannot bear progeny or a son (Delaney 1991, Beller-Hann 1999, Pashigian 2002, Widge 2002). Beller-Hahn (1999) expresses the attenuation of chances of remarriage for infertile divorced women among the Lazi in Turkey. Inhorn (1996: 119) states that in cases when a man in Egypt takes a second wife rather than getting divorced, women consider this as an indication of a man's love for his wife.

The concern for ensuring harmonious relations with the husband's kin also informs the desire for a child. Thiessen (1999) recounts that according to the elderly women in the region Skopska Crna Gora, for full integration into the extended family, a woman should give birth to a child. This is also what the elderly women in the villages where I did research often liked to emphasize. I encountered this issue even more in the interviews I conducted in the two IVF clinics. This concern highlights the needs of women for a feeling of belonging. Single women are 'temporary members' in their natal homes, and childless married women are 'members in limbo' in their conjugal homes. Women 'belong to' the families they marry into. Yet, they do not belong unless they have a child or until they have a son. Belonging is not defined through locality in this sense. It is rather realized by mothering.[24]

It is important that motherhood not only be considered in order to deepen our understanding of gendered ideologies and deconstruct them. An inquiry into motherhood also enables an understanding of what it means for women to have children. Hence the importance of pursuing assisted reproduction treatments.

Before ending the chapter I want to underline a final point. The metaphor of the fruitless tree shows that children are not only desired by women; they are also the means to make women desirable. Nonetheless, despite the fact that this metaphor prevails as a discourse of infertility, in practice, many childless marriages continue without severe marital consequences. Even so, boredom and emptiness may characterize these childless marriages both in discourse and practice.

Notes

1. *Hayır* (noun), *Hayırlısı* (noun), *hayırlı* (adjective) and *hayırlısıyla* (adverb) all mean propitious, something which is meant to be good in the end. This expression inherently acknowledges that only God knows the consequences of everything, so people hope that God lets them experience things with good consequences. Events or things that seem good at first may not be to the advantage of a person in time, in which case they are referred to as *hayırsız* (without *hayır*). If someone wants a child desperately without expressing the wish for *hayırlısı*, the child can be born with a serious sickness or may be problematic in other ways.
2. Kibariye is one of the women with whom I was attending a Koran course in the middle quarter of Village Tepe. Kerime, Kibariye, Cevriye and Ayla became our (my and Elif's) best friends in the village of Tepe.
3. *'Ben nerden bileyim ki, ben tam kadın değilim ki, eksiğim.'*
4. It was not only Kerime who was disturbed by the discussion. The other childless woman went through a more difficult experience, which made her leave in the end. I bring out this incident later in the third chapter.
5. An expression that means he will be blissfully happy.
6. The main reason for wanting a daughter was the preoccupation that a daughter provides. As it appears to me, during their childless years

women get bored at home and increasingly feel the need for a child as entertainment. This is more easily achieved with a daughter because women can occupy themselves with 'shopping for lovely dresses', 'combing her hair', 'adorning her', etc. Daughters are also referred to as would-be friends for their mothers.

7. The idiom 'giving a child' is discussed further in the third chapter.
8. Interestingly, there is also a proverb in Turkish that 'the trees that bear fruit are stoned' (*meyva veren ağaç taşlanır*). The meaning of this proverb is remarkably different from the metaphor described above: successful, productive people incur libel and maltreatment because they are envied by others.
9. Delaney did ethnographic research in a village in Turkey in 1980–1982. Her theory of procreation based on that research has been influential in the anthropology of gender, and since its publication in 1991 it has been one of the most cited texts about procreation. For all of these reasons, I find it important to compare my findings with hers, bearing in mind the time and place differences. In addition, Delaney generalized her findings to Turkey as a whole. So, after even two decades, I find it important to stress those of my findings which support or oppose hers.
10. Here Delaney follows Schneider's (1972, 1984) challenge to the anthropology of kinship. Schneider had argued that the analysis of 'kinship' as a comparative anthropological practice was misleading (because 'kinship' was a European construction), and he had written on American kinship (1968).
11. I will discuss the other aspects of her theory of procreation in the subsequent chapters.
12. In another review of *The Seed and the Soil* by one of the leading anthropologists in Turkey, Sirman (1993: 508) argues that Delaney essentializes culture through a selective reading of data 'in order to prove that all meaning derives from the seed-soil metaphor'.
13. Meeker (1970, 1971), like Beller-Hann (1999), did ethnographic research on the eastern Black Sea coast of Turkey.
14. This is reminiscent of Leach's (1957: 120) remark about the theoretical assumptions in Malinowski's work noted by Strathern (1988: 257). Anthropological practice is conceived as 'model building', and that model contains only the data that 'fit together' and 'make sense'.
15. Interviewed at the South Clinic. This story is also recounted in a similar fashion to Delaney (1991: 76) during her fieldwork in central Anatolia.
16. In Turkish grammar, pronouns and possessive pronouns are not gendered.
17. 1. İşsizlik, tekdüzelik, bezginlik vb. sebeplerden doğan ruhsal yorgunluk, cefa, eziyet
    2. *Bir bozukluğun, karışıklığın sebep olduğu etkili ve sürekli yorgunluk, mihnet*

18. When I left the research field, within two months I heard from Firdevs that she had been introduced to a young man. Six months after that announcement, she was married and pregnant.
19. Kağıtçıbaşı (1982b) in a VOC (value of children) study has intriguingly shown that in Turkey, the psychological value of children is negatively correlated with an increased number of children.
20. This is a popular rhetoric among people who oppose war.
21. The ruling party AKP (*Adalet ve Kalkınma Partisi*- Justice and Development Party) is a conservative Islamic party.
22. '*Yine O Sözü Söyledi*' [He Said the Same Thing Again] Published on the website of the newspaper *Vatan*, found at http://haber.gazetevatan.com/haberdetay.asp?detay=Erdogan_israrli_207273_9&Newsid=207273 (in Turkish), dated 5 November 2008.
23. See for example research conducted in Egypt (Inhorn 1994, 1996), in Turkey (Delaney 1991), in India (Gupta 2000 based on her study in Bombay and New Delhi in 1989–1995, and Neff 1994 based on fieldwork in central Kerala in 1988–1990), in urban northern Vietnam (Pashigian 2002 based on fieldwork in 1995–1997) and among the Han in China (Handwerker 1995, 1998 and 2002 based on research in Beijing in 1990–1991).
24. Belonging is not constructed in similar terms for every family, and the meaning and level of it is subject to change. Belonging to the husband's family may imply the transferral of responsibilities for the woman from her natal family to her husband's family and it may also connote that a woman's primary responsibilities are towards her affines rather than consanguines.

Chapter 2

Religion as Discourse and Practice

In this chapter I examine the pervasiveness of religion in the daily lives of the Turkish people with whom I conducted research. I discuss the influence of religion on the experience of infertility, with an emphasis on the ways in which religious discourse is deployed to confirm one's normality or to avoid suffering. The ways in which religion aggravates the experience of childlessness by reifying motherhood and patriarchal values are examined, as is the mediating influence of religious discourse and practice.

Religious Practice and Daily Life

Early one morning, I wake up to the sound of the *ezan* (call for prayer) coming from the village mosque. It is 5:00 A.M. The village *imam* (prayer leader) is reciting the first *ezan* of the day via microphone to be transmitted through the loudspeakers on the minaret of the mosque. The mosque is a green, two-floor building located at the centre of the village. It has a minaret approximately four metres high. A few men are now gathering in the mosque for the first prayer of the day with the *imam*.

I can hear the sound of running water now coming from the ground-floor bathroom. Selin is performing the ablution ritual (*abdest*) in preparation for the morning prayer (*sabah namazı*). For this, she washes her hands, first the right, next the left, three times. Then comes washing the mouth three times, washing the nose three times, washing the right and left arms up to the elbows three times, washing the ears with the little finger three times, applying some water on top of the head once and lastly washing the right and left feet up to the ankles three times. After that she will dry herself with a clean towel and spruce herself up for the morning prayer,[1] which is the shortest of the five compulsory prayers, lasting about five minutes. She is laying down the prayer rug (*seccade*) on the floor, standing facing the south, the direction of Mecca. She is wearing a long skirt, a long-sleeved blouse and a headscarf, her usual dressing style since she went to Mecca for the pilgrimage (*Hac*), the fifth precept of Islam. She has a rosary (*tesbih*) on a corner of her prayer rug. When she finishes the prayer, continuing to sit on the prayer rug (the last position of the prayer), she grabs it with her right hand and starts to recite the rosary prayers, a prayer for each bead. Her rosary is of green jade stones, and it has ninety-nine beads, as is customary for rosaries: she recites '*Subhanallah*' thirty-three times, '*Elhamdulillah*' thirty-three times and '*Allah-u Ekber*' thirty-three times. The prayers finish when she comes to the last bead. She continues to sit there for at least ten minutes more. She now says her own prayers, that is, her wishes from Allah.

Before Selin, Elif, Osman and I come together at the breakfast table at about ten in the morning, everyone is finished with the morning prayers. Elif and I are in a hurry for our Koran course in Village Tepe. Selin has known how to read the Koran for twenty years, so before we leave, we sit on the balcony with her and read the two pages that are our homework. Elif is more enthusiastic than me to learn how to read the Koran, for she wants to read the whole of the Koran (*hatim*) for the goodness of her deceased mother's soul. This task should be completed before the culmination of the holy month of Ramadan, which is about to start in a few weeks. When we leave the house, Selin will sit down for her own *hatim*, which will last for at least two hours.

Elif and I have a daunting hike up to the middle quarter of Village Tepe for our Koran class. Our headscarves donned for the Koran class also serve to protect us from the burning sun. On our way we pass a saint's tomb. We recite a *sura* (a section from the Koran), *Fatiha*, the usual prayer recited for the souls of the dead, before we continue our stride on the soil road surrounded by hedges of wild berries.

When we reach a cobbled path, we see the mosque fifty steps away in front of us. The houses of our classmates are all around this mosque, which is painted in green. The inside is beautiful with colourful tiles (mostly blue and red). The floors are covered with Turkish carpets. We head up to the first floor, the place reserved for women. We leave our shoes on the stairs and go in. This floor is an entresol, so from where we sit we can see the ground floor, the place reserved for men and the *imam* (prayer leader). Yet curtains keep the ground floor hidden from our gaze. The class for children is still going on. There are seven children, five girls and two boys in class today. Ages differ from seven to eleven. The girls are wearing long skirts with long-sleeved t-shirts. Scarves of bright colours cover their hair. Usually people learn to recite certain *suras* and how to read the Koranic script during their childhood. I am lucky that my village friends are exceptional, as they have left taking this class until adulthood. After the class, everyone rushes to their chores. In the late afternoon, women start going to each other's houses to chat and to practise reading the Koran.

Like childrearing, religion was an essential everyday practice for the women in the villages of Dere and Tepe. People in both villages were practising Sunni Muslims. For the women I met in these villages, religious practices and conversations about religion comprise a major part of their quotidian activities. Most conversations lead to religious propositions, and a great number of the acts performed during the day are religious activities. A typical day starts with performing the first of the five compulsory prayers (*namaz/salat*) and continues in accord with religion.[2]

Reading the Koran, either individually or in gatherings, was a common daily activity. In Village Tepe, Elif and I attended a Koran class with seven (sometimes more) other women for two months before the month of Ramadan.[3] None of the attendees of the class knew how to speak Arabic, but they were all enthusiastic about learning how to read the script. During Ramadan in Village Dere, Elif and I met three other women every day to read a part of the Koran (*cüz*- twenty pages from the Koran). At the mosque in the middle quarter of Tepe during Ramadan, there was *cüz*-reading every day after the noon prayer (*öğle namazı*). After reading the Koran, the *hodja* (prayer leader, Koran teacher) used to talk about Islamic morals. This event was called *mukabele*.

Apart from the above, meetings to read the Koran were sometimes organized to commemorate the deceased or to bless the birth of a child. At other times, meetings served as social gatherings. In both villages, meetings for Koran readings were occasions for socializing and saving money. These meetings, called *gün* (literally 'day'), are widespread in Turkey. A group of women meet once a month in a member's house and bring a certain amount of money or a gold coin to the host.[4] In this way, women are able to collect money to put aside for future use. Since women cannot leave their children at home, children sometimes outnumber women at these gatherings and women are constantly occupied with caring for them.

In both Dere and Tepe, when a baby is a few weeks old, her/his mother invites women (friends, neighbours, relatives) over in order to read the Koran and chant *Mevlüt* for the wellbeing of the baby.[5] This gathering is called *bebek mevlüdü* (*Mevlüt* for a baby). I will describe the event I witnessed in Dere, although the manner in which these are held can vary. The baby in this *bebek mevlüdü* was only twenty days old. She was resting on a piece of pink satin cloth in an elaborate white dress. Her mother, in a white satin night gown, was sitting on her bed near the baby. In front of her was a decorated piece of cloth on which the guests were leaving money, gold coins or small presents. The prayer was held in the living room, which, although it was only 12–13 square metres, was packed with more than forty women. A woman chanted the *Mevlüt* and five women read *suras*. After the prayer, food (rice topped with small pieces of boiled chicken) and *ayran* (a salty cold drink made from yoghurt) were distributed to the guests. The baby was brought to the guests, who held her one by one and recited a prayer.

These gatherings are not pleasant occasions for childless women when children are the main topic of discussion. They are sometimes made to feel unwelcome because of the fear of the evil eye. I had the chance to observe both in this prayer gathering. The women were discussing how to raise a child, often drawing on their own experiences, when an elderly woman sitting next to me asked my age and marital status. When she learnt that I was a single childless woman over thirty, she winced. She cried out to bring a piece of red cloth to cover the baby's face and frowned: 'It is no good to show the baby's face to everyone. Let's cover it to ward off the evil eye'. I felt quite embarrassed and sad, despite the fact that I was not involuntarily childless. I got to experience at first hand the disagreeable situation that infertile women can find themselves in at these kinds of ceremonies.

In the villages of Dere and Tepe, religion helps to overcome the day's emptiness, to a certain extent. If a woman has nothing to do during the day (other than domestic chores), she at least has to perform *namaz* prayers five times, as well as reciting other prayers (*dua*) in the form of *suras*. Sometimes thousands of rosary prayers are recited to make a wish come true, which takes days (or even weeks) to complete. Once a woman has initiated such praying, she usually becomes determined to complete it. In order to do so, she may spend whole days reciting rosary prayers.

Religion fills up one's days and brings joy to one's life – as do children – during gatherings of religious purpose. However, these gatherings are usually avoided by childless women, who are bothered by questions about childlessness and infertility treatments. During one of these Koran readings, a neighbour (who had her first child after she had been married for sixteen years) divulged that for many years of her childless life, she had avoided attending such meetings because of this. She stopped attending these gatherings after a neighbour explicitly scorned her infertility during one of them. Thus, these kinds of gatherings can be a burden for the involuntarily childless woman, whereas for others they are a good occasion, both to say prayers and to socialize.

Popular Discourses in the Experience of Infertility[6]

'Infertility is God-given' is a discourse that prevails in the experience of infertility. Childless women employ it to give meaning to a childless life, to explain infertility, to perpetuate hope, to avoid suffering, to fight contempt and to retain power in social relationships. 'Infertility (or childlessness) is God-given' is a derivative of a basic tenet of Islam, 'everything is God-given'. Sometimes neither of the childless partners shows any physical trait of infertility. This is called 'unexplained infertility' in medical discourse. Nonetheless, it is conceived as 'God does not give', as is seen in the way Kumru – whom I met at the South Clinic – explains her childlessness. Kumru is a 41-year-old woman, who has been married for three years. She lives in an underprivileged district of Istanbul. I was listening to her on a stool next to her bed while she was waiting for an embryo transfer:

> They tell me that my ova are like the ova of a girl of twenty-five which work quite well. They wanted sperm from my husband and saw that he also does not have a problem. So my God does not want to give a child to us.

Women resort to the discourse 'infertility is God-given' in order to bring meaning to their experience. Geertz (1993: 123) noted that religion provides a meaningful framework for people. However – as Asad (1993: 34) notes – he failed to take into account the power dimension of meaning-making in his articulations of religion and culture. According to Asad (1986, 1993), any analysis of religion should involve a historical assessment of power, for it is through power that religion has been defined and practised in the West. In this chapter, I stress that women use religious discourse to empower themselves in situations in which they feel disempowered due to childlessness.

Asad suggests Islam be explored within the framework of a discursive tradition (1986: 14):

> If one wants to write an anthropology of Islam one should begin, as Muslims do, from the concept of a discursive tradition that includes and relates itself to the founding texts of the Koran and the Hadith [a collection of sayings and deeds of the Prophet Mohammed].

For Asad (1986: 14), 'a tradition consists of discourses that seek to instruct practitioners regarding the correct form and purpose of a given practice that, precisely because it is established, has a history'. The Koran and hadith are the discursive pillars of Islam. I argue here that childless women in this research use religious discourse as a rhetorical strategy to achieve certain purposes: attributing meaning to childlessness, gaining acceptance in the social networks they are excluded from or being perceived as complete adult women.

Rhetoric has commonly been used for persuasion since Aristotle. Childless people in this research effectively deploy rhetorical strategies to persuade the people around them about the normality of childlessness. The discourse that God determines infertility, as he does all other sickness and suffering, makes infertility into a common human problem comparable to being ill or being poor. In their efforts to persuade others that they are similar to those who have other problems given by God, childless women use religious discourse. Religious discourse, I would suggest, is more appropriately called 'rhetoric' at those times. I find Burke's (1969 [1950], 1961) contributions on the theory of rhetoric useful for analysing the ways in which childless women negotiate power and identity via religious discourse. For Burke, self-persuasion and identification are key aspects of the concept of rhetoric.

Self-persuasion is a marker of rhetoric in Burke's analysis of the concept. The 'audience' to whom persuasion is addressed was already a part of Aristotle's study of rhetoric. Burke (1969 [1950]: 38) also underscores the conscious or unconscious efforts of persuading oneself as well as other people: 'A man can be his own audience, even so far as he, even in his secret thoughts, cultivates certain ideas or images for the effect he hopes they may have upon him'.

Childless women endeavour to bring meaning to their experience, that is, to have a cognitive framework that makes the situation not only understandable but also acceptable. The women in whose lives religion is pervasive persuade themselves of the normality or even the desirability of childlessness by employing the rhetoric of God's will.

The concept that infertility is God-given is grounded on a *sura* in the Koran:

> Allah's is the kingdom of the heavens and the earth; He creates what He pleases; He grants to whom He pleases daughters and grants to whom He pleases sons. Or He makes them of both sorts, male and female; and He makes whom He pleases barren; surely He is the Knowing, the Powerful (42 Şura [Council]: 49–50).[7]

This *sura* may explain why there is infertility – because God does not give some women children – but it does not explain why God gave infertility particularly to those women. Answering this question ('Why me?') is important in rendering the experience of infertility meaningful. To this end, childless women most often deploy the rhetoric of God's will in three ways: infertility is a test given by God, a reward given by God or it is a God-given retribution. Inhorn (1996: 80–81) notes that urban poor Egyptian women – although they have similar explanations for infertility – avoid asking 'why me?' because they take it as questioning God's will. On the contrary, women in my research asked this question frequently and usually answered it through the rhetoric of God's will.

'God gave childlessness as a test to us' appeared as a popular discourse in the narratives of childless women in the IVF clinics. Accepting childlessness as a test to be endured and staying calm with full faith in God can be called *tevekkül etmek*. Once the test is passed, it is certain that God will reward the person. This thinking thus perpetuates hope. Nurten, a thirty-year-old woman married for six years whom I met at the South Clinic, describes how she stays in *tevekkül*:[8]

> I can say I am in *tevekkül* (*tevekkül ediyorum diyebilirim*). When I think this is God's test, I feel better. I feel blissfully happy, peaceful and lucky. This is a test, which is given particularly to me. If it is in my *nasip* to pass this test [if I can pass this test], it will be wonderful for me. These are major merits [*sevap*]. My God gave this beautiful test to me.

As she goes on, she gives other religious explanations for her infertility:

> My God will give me the best. Whether there is a child or not, I will have the best. Before God, childless people possess the status of the Prophet. They rise to the Prophet's stage in the next world. What can be better than this? There is one more thing. Said Nursi [an Islamic thinker from the early twentieth century] says that in Heaven, one can have a child in five minutes. So, you can have as many children as you want in Heaven.

It is worth adding that *tevekkül* is not a state of passive acceptance, or fatalistic behaviour (Hamdy 2009). As Hamdy notes in her ethnographic analysis of terminally ill dialysis patients in Egypt, *tevekkül* indicates 'constant active and persistent work on the self', 'by acts of piety, such as ritual prayer, reflection, invocation of God, or pilgrimage' (Hamdy 2009: 176, 190). For Nurten, *tevekkül* does not lead to passive acceptance but helps to assign meaning to her misfortune. If she does not lose her faith but prays endlessly and seeks a cure as much as she can (while staying peaceful with faith), God may pity her and bless her with a child.

Nurten's account also evokes the discourse of childlessness as a reward. Having a child in heaven is a reward bestowed by God on childless couples. This reasoning assumes that faithful people who face difficulties in this world will have anything they desire in the next world. The rhetoric of infertility as a reward thus mitigates the ramifications of childlessness.

Nonetheless, infertility is also regarded as punishment. The question 'why me?' can imply 'why am I the one who is given this punishment by God?' The frustration and extreme disappointment of childlessness resonates in the rhetoric of punishment. The perception of the situation as punishment can engender feelings of guilt when women search their past for a sinful act that could account for the punishment. Abortions are a primary example of transgression that comes to mind as a sin that has to be paid for by infertility.

A common discourse among childless women was that 'God gave us IVF, so we can try it'. The notion that Islam encourages the advance of science and its use to alleviate human suffering is painstakingly emphasized in the Muslim world.[9] Tremayne (2006) presents an account of this attitude in Iran, and Inhorn documents the same argument among urban poor women in Egypt (1996), both in the context of the demand for assisted reproductive technologies. Clarke (2006a, b, 2007a–d, 2008) shows that this discourse paves the way for the use of unconventional methods of IVF in the Islamic Middle East such as among the Shi'a in Lebanon. In Turkey, *Diyanet* (The Presidency of Religious Affairs) even opened a hospital in Istanbul that provides IVF treatment for infertile couples. The president of the hospital declared at the hospital's opening ceremony: 'the aims of religion and medicine are the same: to make people happier on earth' (Gürtin 2012a: 297).

Hope

'Everything is in God's hands' (*Herşey Allah'ın elinde*), 'God is almighty' (*Allah her şeye kadirdir*), 'God is great' (*Allah büyüktür*) as well as 'everything is God's will' (*Allah'ın istediği olur, herşey Allah'ın takdiridir*) are popular expressions that convey the hope of childless people. These idioms are strongly supported with faith and narratives about miracles.

Perpetuating hope is significant in coping with the distress of childlessness. As women get older, the need to keep believing in the possibility of a successful conception becomes more vital. Worried about the 'aging ova', or 'old eggs' (Friese et al. 2006), many women in their thirties and forties presume that their chance of having a baby – much less a healthy baby – is very small. Even those who single out medical discourse to explain their fears keep their faith in an almighty God to maintain hope: women can be physically less able over time but God is always perfectly able.

Recurring failures in attempts at IVF inevitably leads to great frustration. Many women who do not want to give up look for a way to perpetuate hope and maintain strong determination. It is usually women who initiate IVF treatments, and it is they who want to go on trying. First they convince themselves that there is still hope, and then they convince their husbands by using the rhetoric of God's almightiness.

Franklin (1997: 192), speaking for the Euro-American context, contends, 'IVF is a hope technology'. According to her, IVF creates false hope for a treatment with a high rate of failure. Promising hope is important in the marketing of IVF. In the Turkish case, hope is still crucial in opting for IVF. But there is an important distinction: for those Turkish women I met in the IVF clinics, hope is not based on the medical technology itself. It lies solely with God. This is conveyed through a popular expression of the rhetoric of God's will: 'first God, then the doctor'. It indicates that God will give permission, and the physicians will then realize your hopes; if it is not permitted by God, the physicians' efforts are doomed to futility. The women I met during my research in the clinics and in the villages would frequently assert that everything is given by God. This approach contests the distinction present (but blurred after IVF) between culture and nature in the Euro-American context: according to Strathern (1992a) and Franklin (1995), the discourse by which IVF is promoted in the media is that nature is 'assisted' by the 'helping hand' of technology (IVF). Culture's intervention into nature thus blurs the distinction between nature and culture.

Women draw on narratives of 'miracle conceptions' in order to keep their hope alive. These are usually God's miracles rather than miracles of technology or science that are found in the Euro-American literature pertaining to the use of assisted conception treatments (Franklin 1988, 1997). Thompson – speaking of the United States – (2005: 4) asserts that 'reproductive technologies may aim to reproduce miracle babies and yet they are so irreducibly mundane. When they work, they make babies and parents'. On the contrary, in Turkey, the discourse of 'miracle babies' is far from mundane. For those women who narrate 'miracle conceptions', it is God who makes miracle babies, not IVF.

Narratives of women who gave birth after many years of marriage are used to maintaining belief in miracles. Saadet, who gave birth to her first child after sixteen years of hoping for a child, is an example. Another woman gave birth to a son after twenty years. Both women asserted that they had their children once they had forgotten about having a child. This implies that, although they had long tried medications for boosting their fertility, their children 'came' when they had already given up treatments. Thus, the children in both cases are miracle children. They are miracles realized entirely by God.

The rhetoric of miracles performed by God is also used to motivate women to pursue repeated cycles of IVF until they get pregnant. People who get pregnant thanks to a miracle share their stories on a website www.cocukistiyorum.com ('I want a child').[10] These women try to convince others to 'never give up' (trying IVF) and to keep hoping. Interestingly, the miracles in their stories are not by virtue of IVF, but by virtue of God. The common narrative is that they achieve conception unexpectedly just before starting IVF, or after failing to conceive with IVF, but never via IVF itself.

Miraculous conception is also found in the *Meryem* and *Zariyat suras* of the Koran. *Meryem* tells the story of a man, Zekeriya, who prays for a child from God to continue his descent.[11] Zekeriya is disheartened due to his old age and his wife's infertility. God answers him: 'Have I not created you from nothing?', implying that nothing is impossible for God. Zekeriya's prayer is accepted and he has a son (19: 1–12). In the same *sura*, the story of Meryem (the Virgin Mary) is also provided. The two stories are powerful examples of the rhetoric of miracle children in the Koran. In the *sura Zariyat*, Abraham is given the news of a son from his barren wife (51: 28–30).[12]

The presentation of IVF by physicians as a miracle was not common in my research. The three physicians I had the chance to work with, two in the North Clinic and one in the South Clinic, would even tell their patients not to expect miracles from IVF. In the media, journalists are more inclined to present news about IVF as miraculous than physicians are. On the contrary, physicians are careful to avoid the narrative of miracles in their interviews in the media. In an interview with a widely known IVF specialist in Istanbul, the physician was quoted as saying: 'There is no miracle'.[13] This, in fact, reflects the perception of the 'miracle' in Turkey, which has religious connotations. By emphasizing that there is no miracle, the IVF specialist underlined the achievement of technology, which they wanted to distance from religion.

In order to cope with emotional distress, frustration and guilt, and to perpetuate hope, women in my research strategically deployed the rhetoric that God had given them infertility for a reason and could endow them with a child in the future. By employing such rhetoric, childless women convinced themselves of the normality and even of the desirability of their condition. They felt stronger once they reframed childlessness as a problem similar to all other troubles (given by God) that one has to encounter in life. The rhetoric discussed above allows childless women to overcome their feelings of incompleteness and become more confident about having complete adult gender identities.

Rhetoric, by providing an effective framework to achieve self-persuasion, is a meaning-making tool as well as a persuasive one. This echoes Burke's remark (1969 [1950]: 172): 'Wherever there is persuasion, there is rhetoric. And wherever there is "meaning", there is "persuasion"'. So far, I have discussed the ways in which women make meaning out of infertility via self-persuasion. I will now explore the act of persuading others. This paves the way to the second key aspect of rhetoric articulated by Burke: identification. Burke argues that identifying with someone is an essential step in persuading that person (1969 [1950]: 55).

Mediating Childlessness

Childless women's relationships with their extended families and friends may deteriorate due to unfulfilled expectations. In the case of a woman for whom a child is essential for belonging to the husband's family, a division exists between her and her husband's kinfolk: she cannot be a part of the extended family. Another division can also differentiate a woman from her friends: she cannot belong to the adult world. She is thus made to feel excluded. Such women, with a desire to belong to these social networks, resort to the rhetoric of religious belief to persuade others that they are one of them. To do so, the women of Dere and Tepe identify with being an adult Muslim woman. Burke (1969 [1950]: 45) depicted persuasion via identification as a marker of division. If there were no division between these childless women and others, they would not resort to persuasion at all (Burke 1969 [1950]: 22). These women employ religious belief as rhetoric in order to negotiate their normal complete adult identities and to 'compensate for the division'. Below is an example of the ways in which childless women use such rhetoric to overcome this division.

One morning, I was having breakfast on the balcony of Nesrin's house, my friend from Village Dere. Nesrin was to be married next week. Some of her relatives, who had come for the wedding, were staying at her (parents') house. At the breakfast table were her cousin Meltem, her uncle's wife Solmaz, our friend Hatice and Hatice's sister Esra. While enjoying our classic Turkish breakfast of feta cheese, olives, strawberry jam, bread and black tea, Meltem spoke about her childless years as a married woman. She had a child after five years of marriage. During those five years, she was considered barren (*kısır*) by her female affines. Vexed by the behaviour of her affines, she criticized their faith in God:

> They say they believe in God, they perform the prayers five times a day. Yet, they could not think that this [infertility] was God-given. That is not real faith. God gave it to me. It was not my fault.

Hatice added: 'If you believe in God, you cannot call anyone barren. It is a big sin to question God's deeds'.

Meltem's and Hatice's comments reflect the way in which religious rhetoric is used by childless women to reconstruct infertility in a positive way and to persuade others of that reconstruction. Meltem was disempowered due to her childlessness. Women like Meltem gain power by questioning other people's religious beliefs and identities. Any scorn about their childlessness will be regarded as questioning God's will, which certainly is a 'big sin'.

Geertz (1993: 119) famously claimed that religion shapes the social order as well as describing it. I have looked at how people shape religion, after Marranci (2008: 15), who noted: 'It is not Islam that shapes Muslims but rather Muslims who, through discourses, practices, beliefs and actions, make Islam'. I look at how religion is effectively shaped and invoked by infertile women. This is most evident in the gendered approach to assisted reproductive technologies. Women and men construct different religions to best suit their femininities and masculinities, and to negotiate with contingencies of power. Both men and women accept infertility as a God-given condition, but women employ this religious rhetoric as a means to gain the power that is usually attained by bearing and rearing children. They construct positive identities and turn the rhetoric against those who stigmatize them. Women go to great lengths to conceive a child, unlike men, for whom children are not the sole means of gaining power, and who employ the same religious rhetoric for passive acceptance of their condition.[14]

Religion and Decision Making

After attending a wedding ceremony in Village Dere, I went to take a stroll and drink tea near the seashore with Hatice and Yasemin, two friends from Dere. When I asked them if they wanted to be mothers soon, I was unexpectedly baffled by their responses:

> Yasemin: Of course I want to be. I will mother a child of an Irish man's sperm.
> Merve: What?
> Yasemin: Yes. When I am thirty-five, if I am single and childless, I will have a child. I will not give it a second thought. I am determined. I have made a thorough enquiry into it. Irish people are noble. I will have a child from Irish sperm.
> Hatice: And I will have one from a Canadian.
> Merve: You, too?!
> Hatice: Yes. I talked about it with my younger brother. He told me I was out of my mind. We can find you a child who lost her/his parents during a war, he said. Yet, I still want it from a Canadian's sperm.
> Yasemin: I spoke to my mother about it yesterday. She was pissed off. She got up at three in the morning just to scream at me. But I am

determined. I have four years ahead. If I am not married, I will have it done.

Merve: I am thinking of adopting a child.
Hatice: No, you cannot do that. It is rejected by our religion. It is *namahrem*.[15]
Merve: Why do you want it from a Canadian?
Hatice: I am not sure. I find them attractive.
Yasemin: Don't you like men with broad shoulders? Handsome?
Hatice: I have never thought of it. Then let it be an Italian.
Yasemin: But there are a lot of gays in Italy.
Hatice: Really? Then, let it be a Canadian.
Merve: Are you talking about your future husbands or children, I am confused!
Yasemin: No, it is important that the child is from a noble man.[16]

I was quite perplexed to see how appealing the idea of having children with donor sperm was for my two friends from the village. They were not involuntarily childless women. On the contrary, having a child with donor sperm was pretty tempting for them. But my confusion was due to my misunderstanding of their desire. They would never consider having a child from donor sperm if they were involuntarily childless married women. The demarcation line was their singleness.[17]

Having a child from donor sperm in marriage was not under consideration for the two girls. Hatice elaborated: 'I would never do that to my husband. I can give my life for my husband'. 'Giving one's life for a husband' is an idiom that reveals the understanding of a woman's role in marriage. Insofar as a marriage is desired, the ideal role of a woman in that marriage is reified. Hatice expects to dedicate her life to her future family, that is, her future husband and children. Despite her strong desire to have a child – so strong that she can commit the solecism of having a child by a means considered unconventional by her family and immediate social circle – being a caring wife seems to be even more important.

The reason Hatice and Yasemin did not consider donor ova was that they preferred to have a child 'of themselves', of their genetic inheritance. Hatice articulated her unwillingness to have a child from donor ova: 'I would not be her mother then. Why would I want such a thing?' Yasemin was also concerned about the genetically inherited diseases a child of donated ova could have. However, this was irrelevant in the case of a child from donor sperm, since there was always such a risk with the sperm.

Not everyone shares Hatice and Yasemin's views on donor ova and sperm. IVF via donor ova is much more common than by donor sperm in Turkey. This is also verified in other research with childless Turkish couples (Baykal et al. 2008, Gürtin 2012a, 2012b, Işıkoğlu et al. 2006). In the North Clinic, couples who needed donor ova were directed to Greece. I was told that demand for IVF via donor sperm was hardly seen. The explanation given to me by the physicians and the nurses was grounded on biological relatedness. Via donor ova, women can feel biologically related to their children through blood (during gestation) and milk (via nursing), whereas in the case of donor sperm, men remain biologically unrelated to their children. Biological relatedness construed as such by childless women is similar to Konrad's (2005) account of ova recipient women in the United Kingdom. The ova recipient women in Konrad's research constructed biological relatedness with their children via the provision of blood (during pregnancy) and milk.

Adoption was not considered among the possible ways to have a child. It was considered to be against the Islamic tenets of propriety, as opposed to IVF with donor sperm which was not. I asked Hatice how she could be sure that having a child with donor sperm was religiously proper. She said, 'It is not written as a "sin" anywhere'. I probed further on the likelihood of its appearing in a book that is over fourteen centuries old. Her response was quite sharp: 'The Koran appeals to all times and all places'. Then she started to recount the facts in the Koran that had since been discovered by scientists. 'Everything is there, you only need to know how to see it.'

In Turkey, adoption is legal.[18] However, IVF via donor gamete is not allowed and is considered inappropriate by the *Diyanet* (The Presidency of Religious Affairs). Hatice and Yasemin's views on IVF via donor sperm evoke the variety of views on IVF. They reveal the creative ways in which religious rhetoric is used. Even views grounded in religious discourse can end up coming to opposite conclusions.

The *Diyanet's* helpline receives many questions about the appropriateness of certain assisted reproduction treatments.[19] The *Diyanet's* website explicitly states that IVF is religiously appropriate (adhering to the tenets of Islam) as long as the required conditions that they list are met. It is interesting that legalities concerning IVF reflect the following conditions in the *Diyanet's* list:[20] (1) The couple should not be able to conceive *in vivo*; (2) The sperm and ova should belong to the married couple undergoing IVF; (3) The embryo should be transferred to the uterus of the woman (wife) who provided the ova; (4) It should be clinically indicated that the operation will not lead to any negative implications for the physical and mental health of the couple and the child.

Recent publications that explain the principles of Islam (*ilmihal*) also include explanations about IVF. Firdevs from Village Dere recommended that I consult *Kadın ve Aile İlmihali* (The *İlmihal* about Woman and Family) on matters ranging from cleanliness to fasting to marriage. The 2007 publication of a similar book (Selvi 2007: 208) includes a section about IVF, articulating the circumstances under which it can be approved by religion. The conditions given as permissible in the book are similar to the ones published on the *Diyanet's* website. Including a section about *in vitro* fertilization in an *ilmihal* points to the significance of 'propriety' of reproduction in religion.

When a reproductive treatment such as IVF is evaluated for its religious propriety, its sexual propriety is in consideration. The discourse on the protection of the sanctity of the family conceals concerns about the legitimacy of the child who will be born to a 'new' technology. Clarke (2007b, 2008 and 2009), who wrote about the concerns regarding sexual propriety in Islam in Lebanon, argues that moral propriety lies at the heart of discussions about IVF in the Middle East. Euro-American discussions regarding IVF with donor gametes concern the combination of substances, which may be incestuous (e.g. Edwards 2000: 234, 2004). In the Middle East, on the other hand, the legitimacy of reproduction with legitimate partners to produce a legitimate child is what matters the most.

The Healing Power of Prayers

There are a few *hodjas* (Koran teachers/prayer leaders) in neighbouring villages whom childless people can visit to seek the 'real cause' of infertility and to get help with having a child (or a son). *Hodjas* are visited for various purposes, such as overcoming an illness or resolving a conflict in the conjugal union. A common procedure is reciting a *sura* over water and having the person with the problem drink it. Another procedure I came across in both villages was wearing amulets (*muska*), which were most often prepared by *hodjas*. Ayla's (who did not have a child for the first three years of her marriage) mother-in-law from Village Dere had brought her *zemzem* water (water from a well in Mecca, which is considered to have various healing effects) to drink, undergarments to wear, and the tongue of a camel to eat from Mecca. Ayla was also having hormonal treatment at the same time. She got pregnant in the end, while Kerime, who tried the same things (the same folk medicine and the hormonal treatment), did not.

Women individually recite certain *suras* from the Koran and pray to God for a child or a son. In online chat forums, some childless women tell each other the names of *suras* to recite and the number of times one has to recite them for a wish to be granted by God. On one of these forums at cocukistiyorum.com, a woman mentioned the Zekeriya *sura* from the Koran, which she said ought to be recited 7,000 times. This *sura* was selected because God had accepted Zekeriya's prayer and had granted him a son. A woman made a suggestion for collecting names of those who wanted the *sura* to be recited for their success in IVF. People put their names on a list and recited the prayers for all the names on the list. They wrote how many times they had recited the prayer for each person. The people at the top of the list were the ones who urgently needed prayers and so each person recited the *sura* for them more times. In this way, the ones at the top of the list reached the ideal number (7,000) sooner than the others. In three months the Zekeriya *sura* had been recited 7,000 times for fifteen people and fewer times for eight people. That a prayer recited for someone else is more powerful than one recited for oneself was accepted by the people who participated in the collective praying. These women subverted the notion of praying as an individual act for women. Praying became a collective act practised by people who knew nothing about one another – not even their real names – except for their wish for a child.

Reproduction Promoted, Motherhood Sanctified

Religion can both attenuate the misery of infertility, and also aggravate the experience by promoting reproduction and sanctifying motherhood to the extent that motherhood becomes imperative (Inhorn 1996). Inability to achieve motherhood, therefore, can have significant consequences such as identity crises, psychological breakdowns and rejection from social networks (both kin and friends).

As has already been mentioned in this chapter, the Koran and the hadith (reports on what the Prophet said and did in his life time) are the discursive resources of Islam. People I met in Villages Dere and Tepe frequently invoked canonical texts and the hadith to authorize certain practices. In both villages the hadith was referred to in order to explain the importance of having a child. An example of such a hadith reads: 'Marry a very loving fertile woman so that I may feel pride over other people because of your number on the Day of Resurrection'.[21]

It is apparent from the hadith above that marriage is advised to Muslims with the aim of reproduction. It is also apparent that this suggestion is given only to Muslim men. Çalışlar (2005), in an intriguing analysis of the Koran and the hadith, reveals that both documents address only men regarding many issues.[22] When reproduction is an important reason for marriage, divorcing an infertile woman becomes grounded in religious conventions. However, in the two villages Dere and Tepe divorcing infertile people was not seen, and marriages usually occurred between people in love.

A few women in the villages advised me to marry and have children, for the Prophet will take pride in the large Muslim population on Judgement Day. Such comments came from people who had heard sermons given in the mosques or at the houses of other villagers.[23] The hadith above also lays emphasis on the fertility of women. This type of discourse, depending on the context within which it is reproduced as rhetoric, can stigmatize childless women when their female affines and friends scorn their infertility by referring to such an authoritative text.

The discourse of reproduction as an imperative act for Muslims was used in a wedding ceremony I attended in Village Dere. The purpose of the wedding was announced as fulfilling the religious duty of increasing the population of the community of the Prophet. The wedding ceremony was a clear example of the reification of reproduction and motherhood in religious discourse, as well as of the growing importance of religion in people's lives.

Hatice, from Village Dere, drew out her desire to get married and have children as a requisite in her religion. Her response is consistent with Islamic discourse on gender and motherhood:[24]

> According to Islam, you should get married. Our religion commands marriage. God alone exists in solitude. You should get married and have children. This is commanded by our religion. The number of Muslims should exceed the number of non-Muslims (*gayri-Müslim*). You know 'heaven lies under the feet of mothers'. I want to be a mother.

Concomitant with this hadith of the Prophet (that 'heaven lies under the feet of mothers'), going to heaven was a prevailing discourse among women in both of the villages. I was often advised about what to do (and what to avoid doing) in order to get into heaven. Having a child is one of the ways of getting into heaven. In addition to the hadith above, I was also told: 'If you bring up two daughters, you will go to heaven'. It implies that bringing up a daughter is so difficult that as a reward one is bestowed with going to heaven. The difficulty is presumed to derive from the need to protect a daughter's physical and sexual safety.[25] Another popular discourse promoting parenthood was: 'If your grandchild has a grandchild, you will go to heaven'. This was more common among elderly women whose children had married at a very young age. These beliefs exert enormous pressure on couples who have difficulties with conception. They feel pressure not only from their parents to conceive, but also from their grandparents, great-grandparents and great-great-grandparents. I encountered only a couple of women who became great-great-grandparents in Villages Dere and Tepe, but it was a widely esteemed phenomenon.

Religion's Reinforcement of 'Patriarchal' Values

When I learnt about Kerime's reproductive history, I started thinking that Kerime was wasting her time with the gynaecologist she was visiting, and tried to convince her to visit another one, someone I knew. He was also an IVF physician, so he knew about fertility problems. I had become an actor in the narratives of childless people; I was now one of those 'friends who suggest the names of physicians they think they are the best'. She gave contradictory responses each time we talked about it. Once she was extremely enthusiastic to try that physician, and the next time she was reluctant. Another day, she said it was Ramadan, she was too busy. I insisted she had plenty of time to make a doctor's visit. In the end, I found out that it was her husband who was unwilling. He had flatly objected to the idea. 'Merve', she said, 'Selim does not want it'.

It had taken Kerime years to persuade her husband to let her have a treatment. Now she felt that she did not have any chance of successfully convincing him to see a new doctor. I wanted to know what was on his mind and I had the chance to find out one day while I was sitting with Kerime, her mother and her married sister in front of Kerime's parents' house. Her mother suggested that I talk to Selim, Kerime's husband, to convince him. Selim appeared in front of us at the moment I was told to talk to him. Kerime, her sister and her mother encouraged me to speak to him. Kerime, with the usual radiant smile on her face, murmured that I wanted to talk about 'going to the new doctor'. Selim immediately reacted by cutting off any attempts to talk to him about it: 'No, I have said no. It is over!' I had to do my best while all three women watching the scene were counting on me: 'Selim, Kerime is longing for a child and I am sure you are as well. I see no reason why you are opposed to going to a new doctor this much. I tell you, he is good'. 'Merve, everyone is good. If God gives, we will have children.' He seemed resolute but I gave it one more try. Luckily, he conceded a little: 'Okay, take her anywhere you like. I am not in it. I permit her to go with you'.

I felt happy that I could at least take Kerime to the physician, but it did not take too long before I realized that I had been misled by my naiveté. No one there seemed to be happy about what had happened. 'Merve, we are not going. We cannot go by ourselves. Forget about it.' It was agreed that two women alone could not make a journey to another city an hour away even to visit a physician. 'We need a man. We cannot go there without Selim.' This was the reason for Selim's 'approval'. He knew we would not make it to the doctor.

I spent that night at Kerime's house. She said if her husband changed his mind, we could go to the doctor in the early morning. Her husband was not even at the house (he works until the morning during Ramadan) and she was not willing to go without him. After the fast-breaking dinner (*iftar yemeği*), we were thinking of visiting neighbours, but before we set off, other neighbours arrived at the house. One of them was a woman in her thirties, a distant relative of Kerime. The other three were elderly women living close by. The women were stunned by the idea of making such a journey without a man. How could we be so insane? Kerime's relative, while trying to make her son sleep on her lap, was preaching about how men and women are created:

> You think men and women are equal and can do the same things. That is a false idea. Men are created stronger to protect us. And since they are stronger, we need men to protect us from men. Women are weak but they are more compassionate. Can you think of a man who can make this kid sleep like me? He would hit the boy, losing his patience. God gave them strength and gave us the ability to mother. *Inşallah* [hopefully, with God's permission] Kerime will be a mother one day. She will be a very good mother. But a woman cannot do without a man.

Kerime agreed with her: 'Everyone is created differently. Merve, you need to learn more about our religion. Come to the sermon tomorrow'. That we needed a man to come with us in order to protect us from other men was the whole theme of the preaching. The elderly women made gestures of disapproval at the idea of two women travelling alone (*kadın başına*). In the end, we never made the trip to see the new physician. Kerime is still visiting the same physician four years after this event.

The fact that she could make her husband submit to agreeing to a treatment shows that Kerime is not a powerless woman who has no choice but obedience. For the last three years, he had been complying with her wishes for infertility treatments. Nonetheless, it is also apparent that his word is the last word. An element of patriarchy is male dominance in decision making. This short narrative makes it explicit that Selim is unequivocally more powerful in deciding important familial matters. Since 'the one with the most say is always a male patriarchal figure' (Arat 1989: 40), 'the Turkish family' is regarded as patriarchal (White 1994: 58). This view underlines the constrained nature of women's authority. A man in the classical patriarchal family – usually patrilocally extended for three generations – has authority over the women and all other men in the family (Kandiyoti 1988: 278). It is the same with overseeing village affairs. In all matters of paramount importance, it is men who are the decision makers in Dere and Tepe.

When it is always men who decide, they are in a more powerful position and their decisions may be to their advantage, implying that gender equality will probably be an irrelevant concept as much as it is an unfamiliar one. In a similar vein, Mahmood (2005: 10) notes that feminism sees the consequence of a society structured to serve male interests as 'neglect, or direct suppression of women's concerns'. In both of the villages I stayed in during my fieldwork, men receive greater inheritances (despite the gender equality in the Turkish Civil Code). In Dere, there was no rule for distributing inheritance among children apart from the principle that men should get more. A man's share was sometimes twice or three times the land a woman inherited. In Tepe, I was told that most often, men had two shares to women's one. The common rule was that women got a smaller inheritance. In most of the eastern Black Sea region, where my family hails from, women are usually denied inheritance altogether, especially if they do not have any sons (though in the case of the lack of a son, men can also be denied an inheritance).

This is by no means all of what I imply by patriarchy. In the context of my research, there are other important issues to be highlighted. For example, the concept of patriarchy makes more sense when it is extended to include the relationships among women as well, such as the relationships between mothers-in-law and daughters-in-law. In other words, in order to understand the implications of patriarchy, one has to look at the matriarchs as well. This is especially true in the experience of childlessness. I will go into more detail about such relationships in the following chapter but it is worth adding here that patriarchy, as I see it in my research, entails the negotiation of power among women in extended families; it is not confined to women's subordination to men.

Another important aspect to note about the women's reactions towards going to the IVF physician is the common acceptance of the idea that women are weak and need protection by men. The discourse on 'protection' restricts women's mobility to a considerable extent (Ilcan 1994b: 567), and this was why, for example, my close friend Firdevs could not go anywhere with me, with another female friend or alone. She had to spend her days in her house and garden with her family. However, she could travel with her nephew, who was fifteen years younger than she was. The young boy had already been given the social role of 'protective male'. I agree with Ilcan (1996: 39), who sees protection as a way of policing women: '[P]rotection serves as a mask for the play of gender and household politics'. Men are granted the leadership of the family under the guise of 'women's need for protection', and this can be grounded in religious discourse, as is seen in the comments of Kerime and her relative. The thirty fourth verse (*ayet*) of the *Nisa* (women) *sura* touches on gender equality in this sense. The first few sentences are as follows:

> Men protect and take care of women. This is because Allah created some people superior to others. Men provide the means of livelihood. Good women are obedient.[26]

I translated this part of the verse from its Turkish translation found on the website of the Presidency of Religious Affairs in Turkey (*Diyanet İşleri Başlanlığı*). There, it is noted with a footnote that superiority does not imply men's importance over women, as everyone is equal for Allah. It denotes superiority in physical strength.[27] However, there is no footnote about women's obedience to men.

In this popular Islamic discourse, men and women are not regarded as equal and therefore need not lead the same lives (women need not work). Instead, it is justice that is favoured (Acar 1993 and 1995). Western women are considered to carry the double burden of work and family, whereas Muslim women do not need to carry that burden because motherhood and being a good wife are roles praised by Islam. This enables one to avoid feelings of guilt for not working (Acar 1993). Islamist journals, by praising motherhood and domestic roles, disseminate such patriarchal values especially among low socioeconomic urban women (Acar 1993).

Kandiyoti (1988, 1991a–d, 1992) criticizes the literature on Middle Eastern women for conflating Islam and patriarchy. This is primarily due to the patriarchal characteristics of the Islamic centres of the Middle East (Kandiyoti 1991d). She notes that those societies were already patriarchal in the pre-Islamic era, and the Muslim societies of sub-Saharan Africa do not show the same patriarchal values. Moreover, she attests that 'classical patriarchy' is also common among Buddhist, Confucian and Hindu societies in Asia.

I find this a crucial point for analyzing patriarchy. It is obviously not constituted by religion alone. On the other hand, it is apparent in my research that the *ayets* (verses) in the Koran along with the hadith, are powerful discourses that perpetuate men's role as the provider and the head of the family, and women's role as the docile, dependent wife/mother.

The ways in which patriarchal values are embedded in gender politics are reflected in a research project conducted with 572 women in Istanbul by Esmer (Tekeli 1992). Seventy-five per cent of the women in this study found it natural that the head of the family is the man, and a woman needs to ask for permission in order to work. Two-thirds of women accepted the traditional roles of breadwinner for the male head of the family, and domestic worker and mother roles for the women. A striking and unfortunate finding is that nearly half of the women thought domestic violence (being beaten by a husband) can be justified. Importantly, the findings of this research also showed that women are taught obedience to their husband by religion.

I have asserted that I do not intend to recast 'gender equality' in a manner that is unfamiliar to the conceptions of the people I was living with. But I wish to argue that religion can be a rhetoric for reproducing men's superiority, and from this it follows that women's roles confine them to worlds in which they enjoy fewer rights than men. This set of circumstances is predicated on God's and the Prophet's words.

Notes

1. The performance of prayers five times a day (*beş vakit namaz/salat*) is widely common, particularly in the villages throughout Turkey. The day is split into five time slots that induce the arrangement of daily activities accordingly. The timing of appointments usually complies with the timing of prayers. A prayer can be performed any time between two calls (*ezan*), but the usual practice is to perform the prayer at the time of its call, which is believed to be more meritorious. It is also worth noting that performing a prayer is not always an individual act. For men, it is a much more social occasion when they perform prayers at mosques, particularly during the Friday prayer (*Cuma namazı*) (only practised by men on Fridays at noon in mosques), as it has a large attendance and there is a custom of chatting outside the mosque after the prayer.
2. The main focus of this chapter is the religious views and lives of the people I lived with in Villages Dere and Tepe. I do not have much knowledge about the role of religion in the lives of the women I met in the IVF clinics. From their narratives, religious discourse stood out as important for many. Almost all the women I met in the North Clinic were wearing headscarves ('covered', *kapalı*), which may be taken as a marker of religious devoutness. However, not all devout people wear headscarves and not all people who wear them are practising Muslims. In the South Clinic, where the socioeconomic status of the people was slightly higher, fewer women were in Islamic attire.
3. Ramadan, the ninth month of the Islamic Calendar, is considered the holiest month of the year. The third of the five pillars of Islam requires fasting (strict abstention from food and drinking as well as from immoral behaviour and sexual conduct) from sunrise to sunset during the month of Ramadan.
4. These are also called *Kabul günü* (reception day), especially when they do not involve Koran reading. See Aswad (1974) and Benedict (1974) for elaborate descriptions of these gatherings in two small towns in Turkey. Beller-Hann and Hann (2001: 162) note how *sosyete* (elite) women who do not go to the mosque organize Koran readings at their homes during the month of Ramadan. It is not necessary to read the Koran in a *gün* gathering, but in Dere the gathering always included Koran reading. See Ekal (2006) for an analysis of the role of mothers-in-law in *gün* gatherings.
5. *Mevlüt* is a poem about the birth of the Prophet Muhammed that praises him. It was written by Süleyman Çelebi in the fourteenth or fifteenth century. It is chanted on various occasions, most often for the

commemoration of a deceased person and in circumcision ceremonies. After the *Mevlüt*, passages from the Koran are usually read and the ceremony culminates with prayers (both in Arabic from the Koran and in Turkish) for various wishes, such as health for the living, peace for the deceased, and for a good future for Turkey and for Muslims.

6. The argument in this and the following two sections was partly published in Demircioğlu (2010).
7. This translation was taken from the Koran database on the website of the Center for Muslim-Jewish Engagement, USC (Shakir). It was available at http://www.usc.edu/schools/college/crcc/engagement/resources/texts/muslim/quran/042.qmt.html.
8. See Inhorn (1996: 80) for a similar account of the ways in which infertile Muslim women in Egypt perceive infertility as a test or punishment given by God.
9. In contrast, this rhetoric is unfamiliar to the wide European or North American literature on IVF. For example, ethnographies related to IVF by Franklin (England, 1997), Edwards (England, 2000), Thompson (USA, 2005), Bonaccorso (Italy, 2009) and an articulate monograph on IVF by Sandelowski (USA, 1993) do not touch on the subject. On the other hand, Kahn's (2000) ethnographic account of IVF in Israel is another elaborate example of how religion informs assisted reproduction practices.
10. www.cocukistiyorum.com ('I want a child') was established by a woman, Sibel Tuzcu, who had a child via IVF. The website informs childless people about infertility and especially about IVF. It gives detailed information about the process, different types of IVF, and organizes meetings with IVF specialists. It explicitly encourages people to seek IVF and persist with it after failed cycles. IVF clinics advertise on the website. Tuzcu has also founded an association called ÇİDER (*Çocuk İstiyorum Derneği* – The I Want a Child Association), which is promoted on the website. The primary function of ÇİDER is to provide discounts for IVF treatments.
11. The story of Zekeriya (Zechariah) is also found in the Bible: Luke 1:5–23.
12. Haelyon (2006: 179) in the context of Israel recounts how the stories of four barren biblical women whose wombs are 'opened' by God inform the perception of motherhood. These stories make of motherhood a 'sacred mission'.
13. *Emir Komutayla Sevişilmez* [it is not possible to make love on command], interview with Dr Mustafa Bahçeci by Elif Ergu, appeared in *Pazar Vatan* on 28 December 2008. Available at http://pazarvatan.gazetevatan.com/haberdetay.asp?hkat=1&hid=13347&yaz=G%FCncel.
14. Men's reluctance to use IVF is discussed in different ways in Chapter 4.
15. *Mahrem* signifies those people that one cannot marry (for example, one's father and brothers). The people who one is permitted to marry

are called *namahrem*. The Koran, in *Nur sura*, verse 31, explains the persons whom one cannot marry. Women do not have to wear headscarves and can be more independent in their relations with a *mahrem*.

16. I was taking a few notes while I was chatting with them. I wrote down this conversation from memory looking at those notes. It is pretty close – if not exactly the same – to what was brought up in the conversation.
17. This reminds me of the heterosexual single Israeli women interviewed by Kahn (2000: 17–23). These are healthy women with no known infertility problems who opt for artificial insemination by donor sperm in order to have a child. This is mainly due to being over thirty, as they are less hopeful about getting married.
18. Among other conditions, according to the Civil Code (253–258), one needs to be at least eighteen years older than the adopted child. There are in total 10,000 adopted children in Turkey according to the number given by UNICEF.
19. Inhorn (2006b: 431), discussing Lebanon and Egypt, emphasizes the disposition of childless women in the Muslim world to seek official religious confirmation of the appropriateness of assisted conception treatments.
20. See Clarke (2006a,b, 2007a–c, 2008) and Inhorn (2006b) for an analysis of Islamic jurisprudence, Sunni and Shi'a perspectives on assisted reproductive technologies and new kinship and Tremayne (2006) for a similar discussion in Iran. See Gürtin (2011 and 2012a) for a discussion about legislation on IVF and religion in Turkey.
21. This translation of the hadith was taken from Bano (2003: 128).
22. See Hatemi (1999: 116) for a reference in opposition to this statement. Hatemi gives examples from the Koran where women in particular are addressed, but he is unable to provide more than a few examples, which is not comparable to the numerous cases in which men are addressed.
23. I have been to a few sermons in mosques and in homes. In these sermons women were told about the 'proper way' of praying (this includes the proper way of wearing Islamic attire) and the ways in which to enhance the piety of their day to day lives. During Ramadan, sermons were also taking place at some shrines. See Mahmood (2005) for a brilliant account of the proliferation of sermons in local mosques ('mosque movement') under the rubric of *da'wa* (God's call to believe in Islam) in Egypt during the resurgence of Islam in the Muslim world in the last three decades.
24. See Inhorn (1996: 83) for an account of the prevalent belief in this hadith ('heaven lies under the feet of mothers') among Muslims in Egypt.
25. The presumption about the weakness of women and their 'need for protection' will be discussed in the next section about Islam's reinforcement of patriarchal values.

26. Website of the Presidency of Religious Affairs, available at http://www.diyanet.gov.tr/Kuran/meal.asp?page_id=83 on 1 October 2008.
27. Beller-Hann and Hann (2001: 114, 169) in their ethnography of the east Black Sea coast region of Turkey, also mention the conceptualization of women's weakness and men's responsibility for protecting their wives. They note that this is grounded in the creation story found in the Koran: Adem (Adam) was created from earth but Havva (Eve) was created from Adem's spare rib.

Chapter 3

Childlessness Among Kin and Friends

IVF assists not only in making babies but also in making parents (Thompson 2005: 5), and so in making kinship (Edwards 2000: 30). Strathern (1992a: 21) argues that IVF assists in 'the making of persons', rather than 'the making of parents' (with regards to Euro-America). In this research, by making parents, IVF assists in making persons whose gender and adult identities with kin and friends are dependent on having a child. It is for this reason that in this chapter I suggest that intragender relationships (Inhorn 1996) shape the experience of being childless and desire for IVF. Thus the relationships of childless women with their female affines and in their social networks are crucial to understanding childlessness. Borrowing the concepts of 'cutting the network' from Strathern (1996) and 'connectivity' from Joseph (1993), I argue that childlessness can lead to women being cut off from their kin and social networks. This inevitably leads to disempowerment and the disappearance (from social networks and from the adult world) of women who are unable to maintain their connection to members of their network.

'I am fed up with neighbours' comments about me' (*komşuların dediklerinden bıktım usandım*), or 'I want the suffering I experience from my female in-laws to cease' (*kaynanamdan, eltilerimden, görümcelerimden çektiklerim bitsin istiyorum*) were frequent idioms in the narratives of childless lives in this research. Some of these women were humiliated, ostracized and made to feel incomplete (as a woman or as an adult).

Not all of the women experienced this. In more affluent and intellectual strata, women's family and social milieu had much less impact on their experience of infertility. However, my observation was that these women comprise a minority of the women who fill the IVF clinics. This was corroborated by my discussions with IVF physicians who told me that despite their economic disadvantages, poor families filled up the clinics. For most of the women, a childless life among female affines and neighbours involved constant negotiation for power and participation in their kin and friend networks.

In this research, the significance of female affines and neighbours to the infertility experience varies greatly from what is found in the Euro-American literature on experiences of infertility and assisted reproduction technologies. The Euro-American literature usually emphasizes the emotional aspects of infertility and IVF treatment instead of its social implications. Psychological distress and frustration due to disruption in the expected life course (Becker 2000, Bonaccorso 2009, Franklin 1997, Greil 1991, 1997 and McQuillan et al. 2003), sexual and marital problems (Franklin 1997, Sandelowski 1993), concerns about the body (Becker 1990, 2000, Thompson 2005) and disrupted gender identities (Becker 1990, Thompson 2005) are all arenas in which emotional effects are observed.

Being a Woman

In Turkish, 'woman' (*kadın*) and 'girl' (*kız*) are imbued with meanings that differ from the English terms related to gender. For instance, the category 'girl' refers to women who are 'not women (yet)', signifying – for many people – that they are unmarried and so still virgins (but expected to marry sometime in the future). Being a 'girl' (virgin) at the time of marriage may signify the symbolic capital accrued by the girl and her family (Bourdieu 2001: 45) who raised her with 'sexual honour' (*namus*).[1] The term 'girl' also shapes the relationships within one gender, between women and girls. This differentiation has been influential throughout my research. Being an unmarried woman, I was inevitably put into the girl category. My 'girlhood', which connotes being inexperienced in matters relating to sexual intercourse, remarkably restricted the topics I could discuss with 'women'. In the clinics, the women I interviewed asked to know my marital status. Upon discovering that

I was unmarried, they would tell me, 'If you were married, you would understand'. This sometimes implied that there were aspects of their life about which they could potentially disclose more, such as their sexual lives. This is a topic that is readily discussed among women, but hardly ever around girls.

This perceived barrier between the women and me was palpable during my research in the IVF clinics. In the villages, I was fortunate enough to make good friends with a few women who put fewer limits on disclosure of information in regard to their marriages or sexual lives. This was also facilitated by the presence of Selin and Elif, who broached these taboo-to-girls topics by talking about their own lives. This usually paved the way for much less restricted conversations. However, my identity as a girl was underlined in other circumstances. For example, when I told women that we were talking 'between women', I was always immediately corrected: 'between a woman and a girl'.

In Village Tepe, where the majority of inhabitants have Bosniak origins and speak Bosnian, *dite* (çocuk in Turkish) refers to a child. A girl of adolescent age is called *sureta*, and older (single) girls are called *sura* or *devolka*. Being an unmarried girl of thirty-one years old, I was considered *sura*. A married, adult woman is called *jena*, whereas *stara* refers to an old woman. The word for female is *jeneko*.

In Dere and Tepe, the education of girls is now encouraged. Some girls continue their education to university level. There are also some families who expect their daughters to give up school, start wearing Islamic attire and be of help to the family with domestic and garden chores. The girls who do not continue their education expect to get married and look after their own kids.

Most of the girls and women in both villages spend their time in the garden and doing domestic chores. They can earn money by working on large fruit gardens for a daily wage. The girls usually keep the money they earn for themselves. The married women more often use the money to take care of the family, to buy new items for the house, or spend it on the trousseau of their daughters. While I was in Dere, the empty building that used to be a primary school was turned into a textile factory. It was rented by a company from Istanbul that produces clothes for international brands. Forty women started to work there, five of whom were from the village. Of those five, one was single, one was married and the other three (who were sisters) were divorced. They worked without an official contract, which saved the factory's management from paying labour tax.

Women's participation in the labour force in Turkey is still low, according to the figures in the Household Labour Force Survey of 2004. 57 per cent of women over fifteen years old are employed, but 53 per cent of this population works in agriculture (Women's Directorate). The high employment in rural areas, however, does not allow rural women control over their lives (Kandiyoti 1989), nor do the few urban poor working women experience this control (White 1994). Rather, their labour is not considered to be work, and does not serve as a social mobilizer to increase women's social status (Kağıtçıbaşı 1982a). Just as labour does not lead to increased autonomy, it does not lead to reduced fertility either, as is the case in Western Europe and North America (Isvan 1991).

In Turkey the main problem with women's labour is considered to be the fact that most women (83 per cent of women who work in agriculture and 6 per cent of women outside agriculture) work as unpaid family workers (Women's Directorate). This means they lack social security opportunities. Moreover, as they are not paid for their work, they do not have the opportunity to manage an independent budget of their own. This seriously hinders women's social empowerment. In Dere and Tepe, in contrast, women could make money by helping others pick fruit or olives, and they controlled the money they earned.

In Dere, marriages used to be arranged by families for their children but now it is more common to see young people deciding on their own marriage partners. However, getting approval from one's family is still crucial. Only one of the four wedding ceremonies I attended was an arranged marriage; the other three took place between couples in a romantic relationship. In the arranged marriage, the girl's (Meryem) consent was asked. Meryem told me that unless she liked the groom and his family, she would never get married. The families permitted the couple to meet so they could get used to each other (*birbirlerine alışsınlar*) but only within the families' presence. As far as I observed, the compatibility of the couple, the wealth of the groom and the easygoing character of the groom's mother were influential in Meryem and her family's decision to choose the groom.

When the couple and their families decide on a marriage, the boy goes to the girl's house with his family. This is called *kız istemeye gitmek* (literally: to go [to the girl's house] to want a girl).[2] After a short period of casual discussion, the girl brings Turkish coffee to the visitors and to her family. The boy's father (or if he does not have a father, an elder male relative) asks '*Allah'ın emri, peygamberin kavliyle, kızınızı oğlumuza istiyoruz; veriyor musunuz?*' (With God's order and the Prophet's words, we request your daughter for our son, will you give her to us?). The girl's father, if it is not an arranged marriage, usually gives a response along the lines of: 'Our children know and like each other. We find their wish for marriage appropriate. Yes, we give our daughter to your son'. Then the boy gives the girl an engagement ring (literally: ring of promise – *söz yüzüğü*). From that moment on, the couple is considered *sözlü*, which implies that their relationship is bound up with a promise of marriage.[3] The father, even if he does not actually imagine 'giving' his daughter away, still uses this idiom as the customary vernacular. In both villages, the girls' relationships with their fathers were often heartfelt, with mutual affection, so a literal 'giving away' of a daughter could emotionally overwhelm the father.

Nonetheless, the term 'giving' is often not totally meaningless. It implies a transfer of responsibility. The parents of the girl, who have done their best to 'protect her' from harm from people (or from men) and to raise her with sexual honour, give the responsibility for taking care of their daughter to the boy's family. The harm is not only expected to come from others: it is also supposed that a girl who is given too much freedom can act in reckless ways that can bring harm or shame to herself and her family. This topic has been extensively discussed under the rubric of *namus* (sexual honour) in the anthropological literature. Bourdieu (2001: 51) explains this as 'negative honour', which 'can only be defended or lost since her virtue is successively virginity and fidelity'. A girl can only bring negative honour or shame (*utanç*) when she fails to act with *namus*. Ayla's mother in Village Dere once told me: 'I have seven daughters. I have seven troubles. Thankfully, I have given them all away, I have saved myself [from trouble]'. This implies that she no longer has to worry about the *namus* of her daughters. Rassam (1980), with regards to Morocco (Fez and Meknes), notes that the need to control women ceases with defloration. I hold that the need to control women never disappears, but it diminishes after marriage or especially after having children in Dere and Tepe.

Within a few months after the *söz*, the betrothal ceremony (*nişan*) is organized by the bride's family, usually in their house. A number of gift exchanges take place during the process of the engagement and the wedding. The weddings are usually held in summer. A wedding reception hall (*düğün salonu*) is rented in the nearby town for the occasion. The civil marriage ceremony is before or during the party. Couples also have a religious marriage ceremony a couple of days before the wedding ceremony. The night before the wedding night is the henna night (*kına gecesi*), a sort of bachelorette party for the bride. These days, wedding parties only last for one night. I was often told of 'traditional wedding parties' that used to last for three days. The elderly women I spoke to in Dere told me in great detail about their weddings, which were 'traditional' and more fun.

Marriage customs are different in Tepe. The common practice for marriage is by abduction (*kız kaçırma*) with the consent of the girl.[4] When the couple goes to the boy's parents' house after the abduction, the boy is praised for his courage and success in abducting a girl. His virility is extolled. Celebrations take place in the house for a week. Relatives and neighbours visit the house to celebrate 'the marriage' (*evlilik*). The religious marriage (*dini nikah*) ceremony takes place within a couple of days and the couple are called 'married' (*evli*). The civil marriage ceremony and party (*düğün*) take place a few weeks later. Couples start sleeping together once they undergo the religious ceremony.

In other places in Turkey, the parents of an abducted daughter may be offended by this act and refuse to participate in marriage ceremonies. Ilcan (1994a: 280) notes for Saklı (a pseudonym), a village in northwestern Turkey, as well as for Turkey in general:

> In any case, its practice [abduction] is always decried. Unarranged marriages show disrespect to one's parents and elders and are considered immoral. As Sirman (1988: 199) remarks, the parents of the bride 'feel dishonoured since the act shows that they have not raised a dutiful daughter'.

Kudat (1974) and Bates (1974), in early essays on abduction and elopement in Turkey, as well as Hart (2007), in a more recent study, also hold that these practices are always against parental authority in Turkey. Tepe, however, remains an exception to such observations and assumptions. In Tepe, where exogamy is an ideal (marriages cannot take place with close kin and neighbours), and where parents encourage abduction, it is regarded as the normal way to get married. The girl's family does not organize an engagement ceremony, but they send the trousseau to their daughter, and they attend the wedding ceremony. No rivalry occurs between the bride's and groom's families, unlike the common theme that prevails in the literature on abduction – referred to above – in Turkey.[5]

In Tepe, men encourage their sons to marry by abduction. This proves a boy's virility as well as relieving the boy's family from any responsibility in the process. It also relieves the bride's family from the cost deriving from formal engagement ceremonies. Moreover, the gift exchange process related to engagement (between the bride and groom and their families) does not take place.

The encouragement of abduction or elopement in Tepe against the model of arranged marriages is noteworthy. Women are not objectified at all in the process of marriage. Indeed, they are able to choose their marriage partners. These facts should be evaluated alongside the facts that marital violence is hardly found in Tepe and childless marriages are likely to continue despite the possible pertinent social hardships.

Unlike the alleged identification of love-match marriages with modernity (Hart 2007: 347, 349), villagers of Tepe whose elopement practices were related more to romantic love than restricted marriages (such as forced arranged marriages), considered abduction or elopement practices conventional. This, as Hart (2007: 350) argues, also reveals that not all rural marriages in Turkey are loveless alliances between families as observed by Stirling (1965).

It is noteworthy that while men are considered to be abducting a girl (*kız kaçırmak*), girls are seen as eloping (*kaçmak*). So, when I ask how they got married, women tell me: *Kaçarak evlendim* (I married by elopement), or simply, *kaçtım* (I eloped). Unless they are willing for it to happen, no abduction or marriage takes place. The first phrase women taught me in Bosnian meant, 'my daughter eloped'. They were not resentful when they reflected upon the experience.

The women who get married are not called 'girl' (*kız*) anymore; they are called 'woman' (*kadın*). Being a woman is almost synonymous with motherhood. A childless woman is still called a 'woman', but her womanhood lacks its essence, motherhood. Being married, but not yet a mother, puts women in a kind of limbo. They are in a constant state of expecting something to happen and arranging their life according to those expectations. Some women in the clinics had stopped working, with the expectation of returning to their jobs once they had a child. An important consequence of infertility treatments is that women have 'lives in limbo' (Becker 1994, 1997 – USA) or 'tentative futures' (Franklin 1997 – England).

Being a 'good woman' entails excelling in one's household duties. A woman is praised by other women when she has a perfectly clean house, takes good care of her children, and keeps peace with her husband and affines.

In Turkey, with the change in civil law that took place on 29 April 2009, women can keep their surnames after marriage. In Dere and Tepe, women give up their maiden name to take their husband's surname, as do the majority of women in Turkey. For my friends from the Koran class in Tepe, keeping their maiden name was inconceivable. In Tepe, even the first names of married women are not used: they are called by their husbands' first names. For example, the wife of Mehmet would be called Mehmetossa. The villagers in Tepe explained that they liked it that way. In a sense, they were proud to be married women, and this practice called attention to their achieved identity. A crucial point here is that they did not have any special names for mothers. Marriage was underscored more than motherhood in this respect. This may be because it is expected that every married person produces a child unless there is a problem. But getting married and continuing that marriage is 'achieved'. Not until a couple has trouble with conception does the notion of achievement in relation to procreation come to the fore.[6]

Female Affines

The anthropological truism that marriage is about families takes on particular significance in this research. In the Euro-American literature, patriarchy has been popularly defined as 'the subordination of women by men'. The domination of men over women has been regarded as a system, or an institution, which privileges men's interests over women, and its reasons have been investigated in biology-nature (Goldberg 1975), capitalism (especially by Marxist feminists such as Leacock 1963) and the state (Lee and Daly 1987). Others have argued that patriarchy predates capitalism (Hartman 1979, Walby 1989, Waters 1989). Some have also inquired into the generational aspect of patriarchies (Hartman 1979, Joseph 1993, Rosaldo 1993), following Weber (1978), who emphasized the dominance of older men over younger men. Recently, the domination of men by men for reasons such as homosexuality (Connell 1995), and in masculinist institutions such as the army (Kandiyoti 1994), has also been investigated.

Within the context of this research, gender politics involves family politics, as the extended family greatly impinges upon the conjugal union. This is the analytical point of departure of this chapter. An understanding of patriarchal domination entails an analysis of same-gender relationships. In the last chapter, the impact of religion in reinforcing patriarchal values was articulated within the framework of gender. Now I will expand the analysis of power relations to include the relations of childless women with female affines and friends.

To understand the domination of women by other women, it is essential to explore the ways in which patriarchy is reproduced by women. One approach looks at 'patriarchal bargains', negotiations in the family for power. The patriarchal bargain is a concept articulated by Kandiyoti (1988: 278), who confined her analysis to 'classic patriarchy', patrilocally extended households found in 'North Africa, the Muslim Middle East (including Turkey, Pakistan and Iran), and South and East Asia (specifically India and China)'. Women engage in a patriarchal bargain when they reproduce patriarchal structures by submitting to their in-laws and cosseting their sons with the expectation of becoming powerful mothers-in-law one day. Women do their best to guarantee the loyalty of their sons who, in the future, will bring them deferent daughters-in-law. It is by having a child – and even more by having a son – that a woman achieves power in her family.

Agarwal (1997: 4) notes the importance of a person's 'fall-back position' or 'threat point' in having 'bargaining power'. She defines this as 'the outside options which determine how well-off she/he would be if cooperation failed'. This is a crucial point in understanding family politics. Cevriye, from Tepe, told me how much she had wanted to get divorced because of the suffering she went through when she got married. She was taking care of sixteen people including her parents-in-law and their children. She had to bake bread and do all the garden and domestic chores under the authority of her mother-in-law. She could never get divorced. Enduring the hardships of a married life and maintaining peace in the family was a compelling social norm in her village. This is also reflected in a popular Turkish idiom: *Yuvayı dişi kuş yapar* (the female bird builds the nest). In the first instance, this idiom may seem to imply women's power. Nevertheless, it is a subtle reification of patriarchal values, such as deference to men. It connotes that when a woman is respectful and deferent enough, there will not be any major problems in the family. I will talk about deference later. Here, I want to underscore the importance of bargaining power. Being capable of divorce and 'going back' to the natal family is important in negotiating one's position in the family. Cevriye's in-laws could dominate Cevriye to the extent that they were aware of the stigma attached to failure in marriage for a woman. Divorce would be considered shameful (*utanç verici*), as women who go back to their parents are thought of as having disgraced their families.[7]

The impact of affinal interactions on the infertility experience is not commonly addressed in the Euro-American literature. For example, in Franklin's (1997) monograph, which contains several narratives from women in England regarding their motivations for having a child or IVF, there is nothing comparable to 'my parents-in-law want to become grandparents' or 'I want a child because I do not want to be humiliated by my sister-in-law anymore'. In the narratives I elicited for my research, such complaints marked women's motivations to produce a child. In addition to mothers-in-law, one's husband's brother's wife (*elti*) and husband's sister (*görümce*) could be a source of anxiety for many women. Childless women who made it explicit that they were never jealous of any women with children would tell me their frustration when they heard the news of their *eltis'* pregnancies. I was told of stories of *eltis* who humiliated childless women for not being able to conceive. Familial power is contingent upon procreation as well as gender and age. Usually it is the wife of the eldest brother who exerts power upon younger sisters-in-law (*eltis*). However, when a younger *elti* bears a child before the elder *elti*, she becomes more powerful. If she has a son, her power above her older *elti* becomes absolute. Being subordinated by sisters-in-law is at least as intolerable for childless women as the cruelty perpetuated by mothers-in-law. Below are some of the ways childless women express how they are exposed to the cruelty of female affines, who may try to end a childless marriage and even start looking for a 'new bride':

- She [the mother-in-law] does not want me. She says, 'let my son stay with me, earn money for me, take care of me'. When there is no child, nothing happens. She said: 'He should take care of me, not her'. She said: 'You will divorce from her'. Think about it. My husband and I were separated for eight months. It was two years ago. They do everything. There is nobody who does not do this [every mother-in-law is the same]. (Nurseli, 34 years old, married for 4 years, male-factor infertility, former accountant-now housewife, second IVF cycle)
- During my first marriage I was living with my mother-in-law. It was extremely difficult. They were being cruel to me because I was the one who had a problem [related to infertility]. She was always saying that she would marry her son to another woman. She said: 'You have not been able to bear a child; we are going to take a woman who can'. Indeed they did. She finished my marriage, that woman. She took away my health. (Hasret, 36 years old, married for 2 years, female-factor infertility, housewife)

– One day, my *görümce* [husband's sister] asked me: 'Are you jealous of your *elti* [husband's brother's wife] now that she has a child?' (she started to cry when she said this). (Elvan, 26 years old, married for 10 years, female-factor infertility, housewife)

Not all female affines make a childless life difficult. Childless women also often want to give a child to very supportive mothers-in-law who desire grandchildren. When the parents-in-law are supportive and thoughtful, women may feel guiltier for not making them grandparents. As Nurten (from Istanbul) says below, a woman may even offer a divorce so that her husband can have a child, and so his parents can have a grandchild:

I have the problem and my husband accepts the situation as it is. I am lucky in that regard. He does not want to see me sad. I am also lucky because of my parents-in-law. They exert no pressure on me. They always tell me: 'my daughter, don't be sad'. They always try to please me. They have never asked me something like, 'why can't you have a child?' They have always told me: 'Don't make yourself upset. This is not the end of the world, you can go on without a child'. Always. As I am the one who has a problem, I tell them, 'let me go, so you can marry your son to someone else and have a grandchild'. At those times she [Nurten's mother-in-law] becomes very sad and starts crying: 'How can you say such a thing? Is it guaranteed that we will have a grandchild from someone else? You are more important for us than everything else'. (Nurten, 29 years old, married for 6 years, female-factor infertility, teacher)

Childless women also feel like they are obliged to produce offspring if their husband is the eldest son or the only son (*tek oğlan*) of the family. The perpetuation of the lineage then depends solely on the offspring of that son. Moreover, the continuation of the memory via grandchildren (Kandiyoti 1988) is also significant for the elders. Couples therefore tend to give up contraception or start infertility treatments earlier than they want to:

When will the mother-in-law have a grandchild? This is always in your mind. (22 years old, married for 4 years, female-factor infertility, housewife)

We did not want to have a child for a few years until the marriage was more settled. However, the elders started to complain: 'we want to see our grandchildren before we die'. So, we gave up the contraceptives a few months after the marriage. (28 years old, married for 7 years, male-factor infertility, housewife)

Not fulfilling the desires of one's affines leads to a failure in realizing one's own self. Childless women's desire to have children is bound up with the desires of their extended kin. Here I find the concept of patriarchal connectivity articulated by Joseph (1993: 452–453) useful in the context of his research in the urban working-class neighbourhood of Camp Trad, Beirut in Lebanon:

> By connectivity, I mean relationships in which a person's boundaries are relatively fluid so that persons feel a part of significant others. Persons in Camp Trad did not experience themselves as bounded, separate, or autonomous. They answered for each other, anticipated each other's needs, expected their needs to be anticipated by significant others, and often shaped their likes and dislikes in accordance with the likes and dislikes of others. They see others as extensions of themselves and themselves as an extension of others. Maturity was signalled in part by the successful enactment of a myriad of connective relationships. In a culture in which the family was valued over and above the person, identity was defined in familiar terms, and kin idioms and relationships pervaded public and private spheres, connective relationships were not only functional but necessary for successful social existence.

For the childless women in the above narratives, their selves were shaped in part by the needs and desires of their significant others as noted by Joseph. The women's selves were articulated by being wives, daughters and daughters-in-law. Their inability to meet the expectations of others severely disrupted their self-images. For example, if being a daughter-in-law and a woman both entailed being a mother, then they were not quite daughters-in-law nor women. Having a child was not only essential to their desire or need for motherhood: it was also essential for the family as a whole.

In summary, the women were entangled in an extended family network. Their emotions were dictated by the emotions circulating in the network. Yearning for belonging prevailed in the narratives of their experience of childlessness. These women described feeling excluded from the families of their husbands, and also from the adult lives of their friends. Without the status of motherhood, they existed in a limbo of failed expectations, living a life cut off from kin networks due to failed expectations. In a sense, their expected networks were severed and fragmented even before they had been firmly established.

Cutting Networks

Cutting networks is a concept I borrow from Strathern (1996). She uses the term in the English and Melanesian contexts to explain how otherwise limitless networks of connections, such as kinship or technology are limited or 'cut' by belonging and ownership. I use her idea of 'cutting networks' and take the following quote (1996: 529) from her argument, but both are reproduced in a totally different context:

> Whether or not accompanied by marriage rules, such procreative relationships tend to share one general characteristic: transactions construct networks of restricted length. Networks become measurable. They are measured by people's indebtedness to one another through the flow of objects, human and nonhuman; those who give or receive wealth, or the people they stand for, become links in a specifiable chain. Claims can be conceptualized as simultaneously resulting from ties of bodily substance and from previous transactions ... Links appear in the chain when it becomes possible to exchange 'different' objects, human or nonhuman, at the point when actions can be taken with them.

This enables me to analyse the significance of having a child in kin networks. Networks are 'measured by people's indebtedness to one another through the flow of objects, human and nonhuman'. Marriage is a transaction that 'construct[s] networks of restricted length'. Once a marriage takes place, a further increase in the length of the chains in the network, or in the width of the network, is contingent upon the bride giving a child to the family.

The word 'giving' (*vermek*) is used deliberately here. Giving as an idiom prevails in the narratives of kin relations. Once the transaction – marriage – takes place, the bride becomes indebted to her affines. In some parts of Turkey, a bride price is given to the bride's family (Canoruç 2005, Kazgan 1981, Stirling 1965). It can also happen that the husband's family asks for the bride price back in the event of childlessness. In neither of the two villages I studied, however, is bride price practised. Yet, even so, the groom's family may still expect the 'return gift' (my idiom), the 'gift' being the money spent on the wedding party and the jewellery given to the bride. Another possible way to look at this is that the bride's family 'gives' (*verir*) their daughter and the groom's family 'takes' (or 'buys' – *alır*) the girl with the expectation that the bride will give them a child/son. Here, the bride who is 'taken' also entails her future offspring. Therefore, when there is no child, the transaction on the bride or her family's side is not completely fulfilled. The bride remains indebted to her affines.

The process of giving is not conceptualized as 'gift' giving. A gift, as Bourdieu (1977) explains in regards to Europeans, is something for which nothing is expected in return. And most importantly, as he also makes explicit in the same context, 'timing' demarcates the European concept of gift giving from the description of Mauss' (1990 [1950]) 'return gift', which is promptly returned. As Ssorin-Chaikov (2006: 362, emphasis original) notes, in relation to Bourdieu's articulation of timing in gift giving, 'with the subtraction of time, the *giftness* is also lost'. Similar to the European context, in this research, 'gifts' (*hediye, armağan*) are not expected to be met promptly with a return gift; that would be regarded as inappropriate, as an act that fails to appreciate the goodwill in giving a gift. However, neither payments on the bride nor on the groom's side are considered gifts. Giving (*vermek*) and *donné* better signify the vernacular concepts. When a bride is given or taken, the offspring is usually expected promptly, as opposed to the delay associated with a gift. Further, rather than the word 'receiving', 'taking' (*almak*) a bride is more suitable. This word also differentiates this type of giving process from gift giving as it underscores an act on the taker's (as opposed to a 'recipient') side, similar to a commercial transaction. However, the giving or taking of a bride in this research was not perceived as a commercial transaction in popular reckoning.[8]

The pressure for a woman to produce a child increases with time. Marriage constructs expectations, but as an act of giving/taking, involuntarily keeping/expecting and returning/receiving (my idioms), it does not ascribe superiority or inferiority to any side. Despite this, the symbolic capital of a daughter-in-law diminishes with time when her role of giving remains incomplete. As a girl with *namus* (sexual honour) deflowered upon marriage, her symbolic capital is higher at the time of marriage. Without a child, her husband, who cannot prove his virility and adult identity via fathering a child, is also under the threat of diminished symbolic capital. Timing is very important in this sense: the other party should not be left expecting the *donné* too long. However, here keeping the *donné* is involuntary, rather than voluntary. Thus the time aspect in this process of giving is different from the strategic time planning in Bourdieu's (1977) account of gift giving. Failing to conceive thus entails involuntarily keeping the item to be given, which in turn engenders diminished symbolic capital for both the woman and her husband. Another important note here is that a mother-in-law may also face such an outcome on her side, for not being able to enjoy the status of being a grandmother. In her case the delay in having a child means not only that her networks are cut, but also her path to power is partly cut.

This last note about the mother-in-law is worth pondering. I have observed that despite their keenness to have a grandchild, not all mothers-in-law are supportive of IVF treatments. I will briefly give the reasons for this before providing a vignette pertaining to a woman's experience with her mother-in-law.

As far as I have observed, there are a few possible reasons for a mother-in-law's objection to IVF. First of all, her son is denied the proof of his virility via IVF. Despite the offspring, the contract is not fully completed (my idiom). Second, in spite of the recent popularity of IVF, there are still many people in Turkey who assume that an IVF child is conceived via donor sperm. This leads to a rejection conveyed as *soyumuz yürümüyor* (our lineage will not continue). It is important that the expansion of the network be secured.

Most of all, concerns associated with social security (financial concerns and concerns for continuing the son's attention towards his mother) predominate among the reasons behind the lack of support for IVF by mothers-in-law. Some mothers-in-law calculate the expenses made for the marriage, for the bride, for setting up a house and for providing for the family. The money spent on the wedding party (*düğün*) and on the jewellery of the bride, for example, in a way symbolizes the value ascribed to the bride.[9] Once the bride is infertile, she becomes valueless in the eyes of her affines, so further expense on her is considered futile. These mothers-in-law are more concerned with their future wellbeing than with their desire for having a grandchild. If a daughter-in-law is not submissive enough and if she is not able to conceive, then it is seen as pointless to continue the marriage, to take care of her, and to spend more money on her. Women can be better off with the full attention of their sons for themselves. The money spent on IVF treatment can be reserved for the expenses of a future marriage for their sons, if it isn't spent on the mothers. In any case, financial concern for a mother-in-law's future stands out as an important consideration in revaluating a marriage as well as infertility treatments.

Sabiha had been married for six years when I met her in the first IVF clinic. She was living on the eastern Black Sea coast of Turkey. She had studied teaching but she was not working. Her mother-in-law was pressuring her son to divorce her and trying to dissuade him from getting IVF treatment. I interviewed Sabiha in the IVF clinic, where she was accompanied by her *görümce* (husband's sister) who disliked the idea of a one-on-one interview between Sabiha and me:

> Ah dear, I suffered a lot. My mother-in-law, my brother-in-law, my sister-in-law, everyone told my husband to divorce. Thankfully, he said he would never divorce. However, all of these people have made me suffer a lot. I had a miscarriage because of my mother-in-law. I lived as if I were in hell during the first year of my marriage. My mother-in-law stayed eleven months with us but I can tell you it was eleven thousand months. I ate blood, I drank blood.[10] I was extremely tormented in that house. She tortured me only because I did not have a child. I wanted my husband to ask for an assignment to another city. Then he was assigned to another city, so we could be saved. His parents even told my husband: 'You will throw this woman out if she does not have a child.' They kept on saying to my husband: 'Throw this woman away, she cannot give a child.'
>
> [At that moment her mobile phone rang. It was her mother-in-law. She had to lie to her about where she was and what she was doing. When she hung up, she seemed very troubled. Her father-in-law had been taken to hospital. This meant a compulsory visit to the in-laws and a total revision of her plans to stay in Istanbul for the duration of the treatment. She continued:]
>
> I went to an IVF clinic. My mother-in-law got into a towering rage when she heard about it: 'How could it be?' Well, why not? She was furious because we were spending money on IVF. She expected me to sell these golden bracelets that were given to me on the wedding day. My parents-in-law did not give me much gold for the wedding. I will sell these anyway to get money for the treatment. But my mother-in-law was raging with anger. It is because of the money we spent on IVF and because of the IVF itself. She imagines that the sperm is from someone else. They never believe that it is my husband's sperm that is used. You cannot convince them whatever you do. I am coming here with my sister-in-law, that woman who is with me. I want her to see what is really taking place here. I want her to learn the facts about IVF from the doctor.

In the context of a childless woman like Sabiha, the links disappear in the chain when the couple does not reproduce. Childlessness 'cuts into the network' and avoids its growth. Even more, the bride becomes invisible – if not undesired – in this 'network of obligations' (Strathern 1996: 524). 'Those who give or receive wealth, or the people they stand for, become links in a specifiable chain' (1996: 529). A daughter-in-law stands for herself and the child she will give birth to. When there is no child, she herself ceases to be a significant link. Connected to her affines via obligations, expectations, desires and emotions, and being partly constituted by them, her presence diminishes when she does not give a child. Further, by not being able to realize her own self, in a way she is obliterated. She is not only compelled to give a child: she also desires to give a child, a grandson. So there is also a 'network of emotional attachments', or in other words, 'connectivity', of which the bride fails to be a part.

Strathern articulates how 'belonging divides' (1996: 531). A girl is regarded as living with strangers (*ele gitmek*) when she gets married. During Nesrin's (from Dere) marriage ceremony, her mother was crying: 'Nobody knows what happens when she is living with *el* (strangers)'. Not until she has a child does a woman belong to the husband's kin. She can be ostracized or maltreated by *el*. A childless woman is thus cut off from both her consanguinal and affinal kin networks as she belongs to neither of them.

Managing Childlessness

What can a childless woman who is cut off from kin and social networks do? How does a woman in such a situation negotiate her place in the network? In order to understand the answers to these questions, I am with Strathern (1990: 6) on the importance of looking at 'how [women] make known to themselves that this or that category is powerful'. In the course of looking at the ways in which the kin categories of a 'daughter-in-law', 'sister-in-law with a child' or a 'mother-in-law' are empowered, I intend to analyse how childlessness is managed by women.

I will first start with 'deference' as a possible way to accommodate the undesirable situation a childless woman finds herself in. Given the habitus of familial politics as has been explained so far, deference can indeed be a valorized way of ameliorating one's position in the family.

What follows is Cevriye's suggestions for her daughter when she gets married:

> Do not expect too much. Learn to be happy with what you have. Respect your husband; avoid talking back. Be deferential in your

> relationships with your parents-in-law; never talk back to them. If you do, you will be the one who loses. Do not exaggerate any problems. Everything happens in a marriage. Do not worry about anything. Nobody's marriage is always fine. You will have children. Learn to be happy with them.

The rhetoric of deference (*saygılı davranmak, itaat etmek*) had also appeared in Cevriye's story about her life as a young daughter-in-law. The way she conveyed deference echoed other women in Dere and Tepe. In the context of these villages, deference is expected from women towards both their husbands and their elders. Deference towards one's husband and elders is reproduced in women's teachings to their daughters and their daughters' compliance with this instruction. As used here, deference implies not talking back (*karşılık vermemek*), not engaging in any disputes (*tartışmamak*), accepting the other's decisions and opinions (*kabullenmek*) and always being supportive and empathetic (*destekleyici, anlayışlı olmak*) even at times when one does not agree.

Deference may also involve asking permission (*izin almak*) for any undertaking (Delaney 1991: 172, Beller-Hann and Hann 2001: 115). The women of Dere and Tepe usually ask permission for daily activities such as visiting a friend in town, as well as for more significant issues such as working as a textile worker in a nearby village. Permission is asked from the mother-in-law as well as from the husband in extended households. The rhetoric of deference perpetuates the relative power of mothers-in-law as well as men's privilege. This was also brought out by Kerime, who described the hardships she went through when she was trying to resist her mother-in-law's demands in the first two years of her marriage:

> My mother told me that I was doing wrong. She told me to try to submit to my mother-in-law. So I decided to give it a try. I never said 'no' to anything she said. I took her with me to my friends' houses whenever she wanted to come. I asked for her permission for everything. When I changed, she changed. She turned out to be a very caring woman in the end. My husband also became quite pleased. He was, before, finding me disrespectful to his mother. He was very close to her and could never stand to see her hurt. That hurt me more. But, when I changed and obeyed my mother-in-law, peace came upon my family. We became a happy family after that. We did not have problems thereafter.

Kerime's mother-in-law decided every detail of her life – for example, making her give up her job as a carpet weaver. After her death, it was her husband who made the decisions. Kerime expressed the positive effects of relinquishing explicit resistance, which had not produced any desired outcomes. Deference, on the other hand, can be seen as her implicit way of sorting out the problems in her life. Kerime started asking for permission or taking her mother-in-law with her, but she managed to go wherever she wanted without any problems.

Docility (*yumuşak başlılık*) is another way of managing familial power relations. Docility does not mean complete deference as always complying with the other person, but rather signifies the avoidance of quarrels while not being too outspoken, by finding kinder ways and times to defend one's opinions. This is what my own mother has always told my sister and me: 'be tender, docile' (*yumuşak*). Many times I have heard from my mother that the way to a peaceful marriage depends on how a woman behaves, that is, her gentle voice and avoidance of any quarrels with her husband. 'Do not talk back' (*karşılık verme*). This is Cevriye's instruction to her daughter as well as my mother's to me.

Abu Lughod's (1990) inversion of Foucault's (1978: 95) assertion about resistance, 'where there is power, there is resistance', as a way to use resistance as a diagnostic of power, may be insightful here. Deference can be seen as an implicit way of acknowledging power, as it assumes the possibility of conflict and suggests a way to deal with it. When the hegemony of men and their mothers is legitimized by the cultural rhetoric of deference, power may not lead to an explicit form of resistance but to more subtle ways of negotiating power.

Deference is not absolute most of the time. Kerime, who praised deference as the ideal way to maintain peace in the family, was not always submissive to her mother-in-law's attempts to prevent intimacy between her son and Kerime. The only stove at home was in her mother-in-law's bedroom. On cold days, a stove was the single means by which to heat the water necessary for the full ablution ritual after sexual intercourse. Her mother-in-law was undoubtedly aware that the inability to have the full ablution ritual would render sexual intercourse almost impossible. This was not only problematic for conceiving a child. As I have seen so far among childless couples (and as was made explicit by Kerime), a fulfilling sexual life makes it more likely for the conjugal union to continue, as it binds the couple. Kerime's mother-in-law's attempt to keep the stove in her bedroom thus prevented the two means for a woman to acquire power: sexuality and procreation (Rassam 1980). After a while, Kerime made her husband buy a second stove, which solved the problem. This at least indicates the relative power a childless woman can have over her mother-in-law and husband. Power thus fluctuates from one person to another, rather than one person commanding absolute possession of it.

Kerime's story obviously contradicts women's demand for grandchildren. The relationships between mothers-in-law and daughters-in-law are never straightforward and I even discovered ambivalence in the desire for a grandchild when a woman was interested in maintaining her son's attention. As explained above, this informed a woman's resistance to her daughter-in-law's IVF treatment.

Another woman, Sultan, recounted a similar story. Sultan is a woman I encountered on a television program where she was a guest. The program hostess decided to sponsor her IVF treatment. I found her number from the television channel and went to visit her in her house. Sultan had lived with her mother-in-law in the first years of her marriage. She told me that her mother-in-law did everything to preclude Sultan from having sexual intercourse with her husband. Locking the door of the bathroom was one of the strategic attempts to this end. In Sultan's case, the attempt to prevent the couple from being able to perform the ablution ritual is more explicit but similar to Kerime's story. Kerime had to buy a new stove, and Sultan had to move to a new house, in response to these attacks on their sexual lives. Neither of them allowed the claims to power of their mothers-in-law to win in their sexual lives.

As I see it, there is a reason for Kandiyoti's definition of 'classic patriarchy', which takes place in patrilocally extended households. Patrilocally extended households enable not only patriarchs, but also the authority of matriarchs, interestingly a crucial faculty in the reproduction of patriarchy. All the women who were living with their mothers-in-law when I met them (or who had lived with them before for a certain time) censured their mothers-in-law for their claims to familial authority.

I do not agree with the prevalent view that the extended family is the desired form as a symbol of wealth and prestige (Duben 1982, Rasuly-Paleczek 1996: 12, Vergin 1985). An important question is who desires it. Instead I suggest that it is the nuclear family type that is preferred by newlyweds and childless women, while the extended family type is desired by the older women who themselves had lived in extended households when they got married, and whose sons are now getting married. The quote below from

Kağıtçıbaşı (1982a: 5) also appeals to a pattern of locality in my field:

> For example, a typical pattern of change through the life cycle of the rural family involves first the newly married couple living with the husband's parents as a valued pattern and due to economic necessities (patriarchally extended family), then moving out as the young man gains more income and autonomy (nuclear family) and then later on, the aged parent(s) moving again for protection in old age ('transient extended' family).

This pattern repeats itself as the young couple matures and marries off their son and when the daughter-in-law moves in. In Village Tepe, where cattle breeding is the main income-generating activity (hence economic conditions are to its advantage), virilocality is more common. In a village of 210 houses, there are 700 animals (cattle). The butchers, as well as other small-scale retailers in the nearby town, come predominantly from this village. However, like Cevriye, villager women see that fewer sons stay with their parents today. Cevriye's two married sons live in the nearby town, whereas she lived with her parents-in-law for sixteen years.

A radical response to a life made difficult by living with female affines is moving to a new house. In the IVF clinics I met childless women who had convinced their husbands to move out. As I was told by two women, it was not easy to manage their in-laws and husbands in this process, but once they were determined, they could succeed in setting up an independent household.

The discourse most common among mothers-in-law (in Dere and Tepe) about daughters-in-law is that *şimdiki gelinler* (daughters-in-law of today) are different. The saying *Şimdi kaynanalar gelin, gelinler kaynana oldu* ('Today mothers-in-law have become daughters-in-law and daughters-in-law have become mothers-in-law') reflects the subversion in family politics today. Mothers-in-law bemoan their daughters-in-law for not being submissive, for not taking good care of their mothers-in-law (and of their sons) and for moving to independent households. Most daughters-in-law complain about how their mothers-in-law whine about them to their husbands. In a discussion I had in Village Dere with elderly mothers-in-law, they had the same complaint about their daughters-in-law. One of them said: 'A rat has come to our house, who uncovers our thing [vagina], who writes all the day and reads all the night'.[11] This was met with both laughter and seriousness. The acceptance of the analogy of a rat for a daughter-in-law among women gives another clue to the animosity harboured towards daughters-in-law of today. Outspoken and disobedient daughters-in-law are especially disliked. 'Writing all day and reading all night' implies that some daughters-in-law spend the day looking for complaints to make to their husbands about their mothers at night. Keeping everything secret, especially incidents with one's mother-in-law, is highly praised. *Kol kırılır, yen icinde kalır* (the broken arm stays inside the sleeve) is a proverb that reifies such secrecy. This proverb also indicates valorization of concealing familial or marital problems. Having a disobedient daughter-in-law is similar to not having a daughter-in-law (because of not having a son), in the sense that what was 'bargained for' cannot be enjoyed now.

The discourse on the part of mothers-in-law about changes in the relationship between powerful mothers-in-law and submissive daughters-in-law has been elaborated by Kim (1996) and Vera-Sanso (1990), for South Korea and southern India respectively. Kim sees these relationships in the family in the form of a triadic relationship among the wife, the husband and the husband's mother. She admits that in South Korea, the mothers-in-law of today are called the 'double-loss generation', as they experienced hardship from their mothers-in-law when they were young, and now they are experiencing hardship from their daughters-in-law.

On the other hand, I do not hold that the power balance has been reversed from a prior state. My sense of familial relations from my research suggests a more itinerant relationship. Ongoing negotiations of power have a continuous impact on power balances. Vera-Sanso (1990) bases these relationships on expectations, fear of the future and current circumstances, which also apply to my research. Simic (1983) articulates the family dynamics in the cultural arena of former Yugoslavia in the form of three dyadic relationships: husband/wife, mother/son and daughter-in-law/mother-in-law. Whether three dyads or one triad (Kim 1996), these are various conceptual tools for looking at the same thing, which end up making similar claims: the undeniably powerful presence of the mother-in-law in the life of the conjugal unit, and the challenge it creates for the daughter-in-law.

The Conjugal Union

Before going into the relationships between childless women and their neighbours, I want to underscore a few observations in regards to husband-wife relationships. In order to elucidate the influence of affines on childless women, I focused on the nature of their relationships. I prioritized the female affinal relationships over the conjugal union as this was consistent with how the women I interviewed described their experience of being childless. Unless I asked, husbands rarely appeared in women's narratives. Nevertheless, I make a final note about the nature of involuntarily childless conjugal unions.

As I said, women did not often bring up their husbands in their narratives. When they did, it was predominantly about the supportive nature of their husbands. Yet one woman told me that she had suffered because her husband did not mediate her relationship with his parents. Another woman from the Black Sea region complained about husbands who divorced their wives and took a second wife in the case of childlessness. A woman from Istanbul said her husband ostracized her. Except for those three, the women I encountered in the IVF clinics liked to emphasize the support and kindness they received from their husbands.

Inhorn's (1994, 1996) research about infertile couples in poor urban Egypt emphasizes the love and attachment that binds couples in childless marriages despite the social suffering faced within the extended families. Unlike the strictly gender-segregated and functional marriages (in which husband and wife are only together to produce and rear a child) devoid of affect between the husband and wife described by Mernissi (2003 [1975]) for Muslims, my research showed that love, care, support and friendship were important for the married couples. Childlessness does not necessarily injure marital relationships. Sometimes 'sharing a problem' was mentioned as a cause binding the couple to each other. Feelings of caring for each other and gratefulness for each other's support also seem to have positive implications for some childless marriages.

This rhetoric of 'support' (*destek*), however, needs some clarification. Some of the women used the term as an analogy for their husbands' efforts to 'protect' their wives from their female affines. Some of them called their husbands supportive for not always complying with their mother's wishes. Others used it to imply that their husbands consented to treatment. It most often implied that the husband 'did not make infertility a huge problem'. It implied they provided emotional support to ease the minds of their wives, who were preoccupied with infertility: 'He tells me that it is not the end of the world'. Sometimes support was not achieved from doing something but instead from not doing a particular thing, such as pressuring, humiliating or threatening. In a few cases, it was taking over the blame of infertility so that nobody could disparage the woman. However, this was extremely rare because of the stigma attached to male infertility.

There were also times when I had doubts about this 'support'. Women would sometimes tell me how supportive their husbands were because they were being very thoughtful and not talking about having a child. These husbands' love for children is apparent in the extreme affection they show to the children of other people: 'My husband loves children so much' that 'he always hugs our neighbour's three-year-old kid', 'he buys other children gifts' or 'he plays with his brother's child for a long time, with great patience'. Women feel more envious in those cases and more distressed for not being able to give a child to their husbands. When I heard these stories, I was not sure whether the husbands were sending a subtle message to their wives by cuddling babies and toddlers. It seems unlikely to me that men do not think of what their infertile wives would feel when they see their husbands 'dying for a child'.

An important remark should be made about the guilt that is felt for the other partner because of childlessness. Since I have interviewed women, my observation with regards to the gendered nature of this guilt is limited. All the women with fertility problems I interviewed expressed feelings of guilt for 'not making their husbands fathers' (*kocalarını baba yapamamak*). There were also a few women who told me how sad their infertile husbands were because of not making their wives mothers. But the general consensus was that – despite the discourse of the supportive husband – wives of infertile men are more caring and thoughtful than the husbands of infertile women, and there are fewer cases of divorce in the case of male infertility.

It is worth noting that polygamous marriages, or having a *kuma* (concubine, second wife), do exist in Turkey despite their illegality – although they are not found in Dere or Tepe. A man can marry a second woman via a religious marriage ceremony.[12] In their social circles, these couples can be considered married. If a man's first wife is married to him only via a religious ceremony, in other words not legally married, he can get married to another woman via a civil ceremony, in which case the first wife falls into a precarious position. The infertile first wife in that case has no economic security. If her husband dies, only the legally married wife and her children will receive inheritance. If the second woman from whom a man has children is married to him only via a religious ceremony, her children will still receive inheritance upon the man's death. A woman with children thus has a more financially advantaged and secure position.

Neighbours

Neighbours exert enormous control over people's lives.[13] This is not only valid for those in Dere and Tepe. The influence of neighbours on the experience of infertility dominated the narratives of childless women I met in the IVF clinics. The intensity of neighbours' control increases over the course of childless women's lives. Being childless has a drastic effect on the balance of power in the relationships among neighbours. Women with children, as I see it, acquire a more powerful position from which they deem themselves superior. They probe the lives of childless women through a myriad of questions, and this knowledge is then used for supporting, criticizing, humiliating or counselling.

Quarters (*mahalle*) in the villages of Dere and Tepe are regarded as neighbourhoods. One's neighbours are usually those who live in the same quarter. In Tepe, unlike the village of Dere, exogamy is the rule for marriage. Marriage prospects can never be kin or a neighbour from the same quarter. For instance, in Tepe, the fifth generation descendants of two brothers are considered 'too close' (*fazla yakın*) to get married.[14] Cevriye's and Kibariye's children are in this situation of being considered close kin. Thus, Cevriye's daughter can never be a marriage prospect for Kibariye's son. The patrilineage is not necessarily invoked to claim closeness. The grandchildren of sisters cannot marry either. Exogamy is not confined to blood-relatedness. The proximity of the houses leads to 'closer' neighbourhoods. The villagers in the 'middle quarter' of the village Tepe also consider themselves 'too close' to let their children intermarry. Kerime's family is not related to Cevriye's or Kibariye's families by blood. Yet I was told that if she had a child, her child's marriage into Cevriye's or Kibariye's families would not be possible. However, these people can marry their children to villagers from other quarters, provided that they are not kin. Edwards and Strathern (2000: 151) note: 'A claim on the place entails a claim on those that belong to the place'. In Tepe the claim on those people who belong to the middle quarter prevents marriage among them.

The female inhabitants of a quarter usually have complete knowledge of what is going on in each other's lives. The 'middle quarter' where my friends lived is such a quarter. They have many chances to spend time together during the day, such as helping one another with baking, or reading the Koran. After supper, going to each other's houses with needlework in a plastic bag is the custom. Women prefer that their husbands go to the village *kahve* (local coffee shop for men), which leaves women the freedom to go anywhere they like. When the husbands do not go to the coffee shop, home visits are made as couples. Women usually chat while doing embroidery and drinking tea. During these visits hosts and visitors are not necessarily segregated by gender.

As Edwards (2000: 220) writes in the context of her research in Bacup, England: 'The other face of being close, however, is being too close. The close-knit community, for example, is both a source of support and gossip'. Hatice from the village of Dere often complains about the overly close nature of relationships in the village and about the immense amount of knowledge the villagers have about her. 'The women I greet on the street knew me even as a baby. They knew my school years as a child. There is nothing they do not know about me. I am bored stiff.' She is also tired of the neighbours who still interrogate her about why she is not yet married. Hatice is so wearied by people's involvement in her life and the pressures they put on her that she wants to leave the village for a metropolis like Istanbul, where 'nobody knows and cares about one other'. 'Istanbul is like Heaven. You can walk on the streets among millions of people who do not know you. They do not care if you are married or not.' Differentiation of the city (a place where one may preserve one's anonymity) from the village (a place where everyone claims an interest in one's personal business) echoes the distinction made between urban and rural environments by the residents of Bacup in Edward's (2000: 240) research. However, by Hatice's reckoning, the anonymity of the city is not 'cold' or characterized by 'utilitarian relationships', but has positive connotations, specifically freedom from social constraints and expectations.

Hatice has refused to marry the prospective grooms to whom she has been introduced because she says she wants to be 'selective' (*seçici*). However, she feels compelled to marry as soon as possible just because she does not want to hear any more reproaches about her celibacy. Hatice is among countless people who complain about other people's interference in their lives and who have to align their lives with the expectations of others. It is not uncommon for people to be asked about when they are going to get married, the reasons for their celibacy and when they are going to have children. If they do not have children, people are asked if they have been to a physician, if they are under any treatment, if they have tried some local medicine, if they have visited a hodja, 'who has a [fertility related] problem', if they are having protected sex, and even sometimes if their husbands are 'male'. These are only a few of the questions that people face in their everyday lives. One woman in Tepe put it clearly: 'When you are growing up, you are your parents' trouble. When you are grown up, your life troubles everyone'.

Cohen's (1982: 10–11) argument about the publicness of knowledge is illustrative in this context. In small-scale societies, he remarks, all kinds of knowledge about people are salient, public and indivisible parts of social relationships. The public nature of personal information compels people to be careful about the disclosure of knowledge, and to 'accord with conventions', which can at times, cause tension. He argues, furthermore, that the publicity of knowledge is 'an essential currency for social interaction'. It is indeed apparent in Hatice's case that she experiences tension from trying to conform to social expectations.

An experience of Kerime's is a case in point. Kerime's menstrual period was delayed when we were attending the mosque every day during the month of Ramadan. Unless a woman has her menstrual period, she continues to go to the mosque, and Kerime continued to attend for the whole month. Everyone was aware of the delay in Kerime's menstrual period. All the women who saw her asked whether she was pregnant. This made her believe more in her pregnancy. Her excitement was visible in her eyes and smiling face. In her absence, women continued to talk about it: 'We did not know that Kerime and her husband wanted it so much. Selim [Kerime's husband] does not let her travel anywhere. He has become very caring. Apparently he is also desperate for a baby'. There was intense gossiping going around about the delay in Kerime's menstrual period and about their 'keenness' to have a baby. It became obvious that they were not able to have a child despite their strong desire for one. It was one of the hardest times of her life when Kerime had her period after six weeks.

Kerime and Selim's experience is reminiscent of what Goffman calls 'stigma management', which is 'the management of undisclosed discrediting information about self' (1963: 42). Goffman's argument about stigma management has been criticized by Riessman (2000a, 2000b) who did research in Kerala, South India. Riessman indicates that stigma management is not applicable to the childless people in non-Western settings where voluntary childlessness is not common. Since voluntary childlessness is nearly inconceivable in most places, childless women are always considered infertile. This critique of stigma management applies to the experience of Kerime described above. Inhorn (1996: 186, 205), speaking about Egypt, also remarks that information management is not a straightforward issue with regards to infertility, although it is possible. One's consanguines help childless women control the degree and type of information conveyed to others. In Tepe, where Kerime lives, nondisclosure of infertility is almost impossible, especially after a few years of married life.

For women, enquiries about marriage and having children are more troubling because of the immense urge they generate for people to know why a woman has not accomplished these things yet. This is not only true in the villages, nor is it confined to the working class. I was lucky to meet a woman in the second IVF clinic, Suna, with whom I made good friends. Suna had not disclosed her treatment to anyone. She wanted to avoid the myriad questions she would have to face, were she to tell anyone. Endless enquiries by 'other people' (*başkaları, çevre*) about her life had a considerable impact on the decisions she had made. In her mid-twenties she was already annoyed by the questions she faced about marriage, so she married:

> I told myself that if there was a decision made for me to marry, I would concede. I wanted to silence everyone. In a year, I realized that I would never be able to silence anyone, but I was already married. I experienced every sort of problem one could go through during marriage, but I did not want to give up, and I managed to overcome them one by one. I had only one choice: to make a go of it ... I could end my marriage but what would have happened then? Then all those thousands of voices would appear again: 'Did you divorce?' 'She *could not* continue her marriage.' 'Who is she going to marry now?' I cannot close my ears to these voices because I have a mother and a sister.

Suna was a university graduate with a promising career in business and a wealthy family. Her narrative reveals that the anxiety induced by the involvement of others in one's life cuts across social classes. People are not only born into – or married into – a set of social roles among family members. Roles also have to be played out in circles of friends and acquaintances. Suna felt the anxiety of meeting people's expectations for her marriage. Once she is married, she is obliged to continue that marriage and to have a child as well. Divorce would be a failure that would humiliate her.

Enquiries about other people's lives are more common among women than men. Marriage and children are popular subjects among women, putting single or childless women in a much more difficult position than their male counterparts. It is the childless women whose lives are investigated and interfered with most. The control of knowledge and (reproductive) practices among women does not dramatically affect their lives if they are on the same terms, i.e. if they are all married and have sons. Below are a few examples of the influence of neighbours on the decision to conceive a child:

- Neighbours are very difficult to cope with. They decide your lifestyle. They put you in depression. You cannot just say, 'I do not want to have a child'. You *have to do it* in the end. It is like everyone is managing your life with invisible ropes. (42 years old, married for 6 years, female-factor infertility, nurse, sixth IVF cycle)
- We did not want to have a child in the beginning because I was too young. But everyone asked so many questions about it that we felt pressure on us. So we decided to visit a doctor. (38 years old, married for 22 years, female-factor infertility, housewife, has a son)
- My neighbours pressure me a lot. They tell me to have IVF. They found a job with social security for my husband. They think they are a great support. I can never tell them the truth; it is very difficult. (35 years old, married for 15 years, vaginismus, housewife)[15]

The narratives evoke the control people exercise on the lives of childless women. Sometimes they provide support; sometimes they radically influence the plans of childless women by inducing them to initiate conception or treatment before they had planned. The woman above faces even more pressure because she cannot tell her neighbours the truth, that her 'problem' is vaginismus. She finds it hard to make up answers to the countless questions about her 'problem'.

Dealing with interrogations about childlessness – stigma management – is not an easy task. During the first years of marriage, childlessness is presented as voluntary. Women complain about the guilt they feel about 'lying to people', about misrepresenting their intentions, and for concealing their fertility treatments. But the situation is even more difficult after a few of years of marriage (or a few months or even weeks for some people), when it is assumed that they are involuntarily childless. The types of questions are altered due to this assumption. Sometimes women are advised to visit a physician and are given names of physicians. They are told not to worry about it and are provided with examples of people who finally conceived after years of marriage. At other times they are humiliated because of their failure to conceive. The question of 'Whose fault is it?' (*Problem/sorun kimde? Kimin suçu?*) is always of interest. Men's alleged fault in conception due to sexual impotence is an insult harder to cope with. Women, sometimes, are told to adopt a child. This is taken as an insult, particularly when it is a female in-law telling them to adopt. In this sort of adoption, the recommendations are usually scornful: 'If you want, I can make one and give her/him to you' (*istersen ben sana yapıp bir tane vereyim*), 'let your sister-in-law make and give one to you' (*görümcen yapıp sana versin*). Women are also disturbed by the comparisons made with other women who got married at the same time but who now have children. 'She married at the time you did, but she has many children' (*'Seninle evlendi, kaç çocuğu var'*).

Childless women resent questions that cross the boundaries of privacy. Sometimes they are asked about their sexual life, how they are protected, and so on. As one woman in the South Clinic put it: 'They ask me questions about my bedroom. Do they need to know everything only because I do not have a child?' This is a crucial point. Women may not ask such questions of women with children. Yet, they feel they have a right to ask personal questions of childless women. As if she is a physician asking about a patient's sexual life, a woman with a child claims enough power or knowledge (Foucault 1977, 1978, 1980) to see herself as an expert on producing a child only because she herself has done so. Edwards (2000: 34), discussing the people she met in Bacup, notes: 'It is their experience of kinship which qualifies them to speak with authority about ART'. It is as if women with children claim a position of authority on procreation, since they have been able to do so at least once. 'Have you tried giving your husband carob?' is an example of a question that is also a subtle contestation of the childless man's sexual potency.[16] Having a child renders a woman more powerful in such social interactions. Not having had a child, a woman's life can be controlled by other women who 'know how to have a child' or who 'were able to produce a child'.

Childless women are made to feel incomplete and inferior through the assumption that they cannot understand certain things because of their childlessness. In Village Tepe, while I was having a discussion in Kibariye's home about having children with my friends from the Koran class and a few of their friends, I encountered a similarly frustrating experience. Arzu had entered into menopause without having children. She was telling us that she loves Kibariye's children so much that she feels like a mother to them. Everyone in the group made caustic remarks to her about this, saying that she could never understand what it means to be a mother without being one. When she said, 'Every woman is born a mother, I read it somewhere', she was told not to believe everything she read. Arzu tried to assert her mother-woman identity against women who relentlessly deemed her inferior, as somehow incomplete. Childless women usually emphasize their distress over being put in an inferior position where it is assumed they know less than others and always will. 'Not knowing' not only involves the emotions and practices pertaining to motherhood; it also signifies that women who are not mothers are not capable of understanding everything. This is because they are not grown up enough to acquire full adult identities yet. Procreation appears to be a prerequisite for achieving one's full adult identity. Below is a pertinent example, elicited during an interview I had with Nehir, at the South Clinic. Nehir is thirty years old and has been married for six years. She is a high school graduate and her husband, who has an impressive career in freight, has a postgraduate degree. They live in a privileged part of Istanbul:

> There is only one thing that distresses me. When I am told, 'you cannot understand this, you do not have a child', I feel very sad. Do you need to have a child to understand things? ... People with children think that they are more capable of understanding everything only because they have a child. We too, can understand.

In order to avoid such interactions, some childless women avoid gatherings with other women; they tend to socialize less as time goes by. They also give up visiting the homelands of their parents and their husbands, which are sometimes small villages in Anatolia where everyone knows and enquires about each other. As time passes, when the disclosure of involuntary childlessness is inevitable, they can be marginalized, being voluntarily asocial, or worse, ostracized. They are cut off from their social networks, as a couple of vignettes I elicited in the IVF clinics illustrate:

- Being childless is awful. You are offended in social gatherings. Women touch your belly and ask 'Not yet?' You do not want to be among people. You do not want to be seen as inferior [*aşağı görülmek*]. You cannot socialize at all. This is unexplainable. It is horrible. (31 years old, married for 10 years, female-factor infertility, housewife, second IVF cycle)

- I cannot go to *mevlüts* for babies. Everyone talks about children. The most terrible thing is that people think you will cast the evil eye on them or on their children. I cannot decide where to look. They never give me the babies for praying as if harmful rays spread out from me. They think their children are perfect but they are not. But, you know, it is only a child in the end. The difference, my dear, is that they were able to have that child but I was not. That is a big difference among us. (37 years old, married for 11 years, male and female infertility, housewife, second IVF cycle)
- When you are hurt outside, you want to run home. You are happy only at home. (Nesrin's [from Dere] cousin who succeeded in having a child only after five years of marriage)

These narratives demonstrate the difference that a child can bring to a woman's social relationships. Conceiving a child is a prerequisite for being a participant in a social network of friends who have more or less equal power claims to each other. When the women above attempt to be a part of that network, they are reminded of what they lack, whether this is children or the capacity to understand certain things. They are also sometimes reminded of something their husbands allegedly lack: sexual prowess. Failure to conceive puts these women in such an inferior and unbearable position that they have no choice but to be cut off from the network until they achieve conception.

Stereotyping is another form of castigating childless women, which forces them to be cut off from social networks. As was discussed in the first chapter, childless women are frequently called 'trees that do not bear fruits'. They are also called 'dry', which is a direct reference to infertility (and to dry trees). There are also a few other epithets popularly ascribed to childless women such as cruel (*zalim*), merciless (*acımasız*), stingy (*cimri*) and insensitive (*anlayışsız*). The word used for infertile or barren, *kısır*, is itself humiliating and disturbing enough for the childless women.

For men, the stereotypes are directly linked to their male identity. *Erkek değil* (not male) is the most offensive stereotype, while being *zürriyetsiz* (without progeny) is also upsetting.[17] Stereotyping usually occurs between women with children and childless women. Even the terms about men are used by women with children in conversation with childless women. It is quite rare that this kind of humiliation happens between men and women. Among men, children as a subject is not much discussed, let alone childlessness.

It was made explicit by some women in Tepe that men avoided making direct remarks about childlessness in order to avoid fights.

In conclusion, I can argue that intragender relationships inform the infertility experience for both women and men, and having a child becomes an obligation for rendering the publicly accepted roles of being a wife and a daughter-in-law. Cohen (1982: 10, 1994) argues against the use of 'social roles' as a useful concept in anthropology. He claims that the replacement of role with self in most anthropological analysis renders people partial and precludes seeing the agency and creativity of whole people engaged in their social interactions. I do not agree that an analysis that makes use of 'social roles' shows people as fatalistic beings with no agency. I have shown throughout this chapter that social roles become a source of anxiety with regard to one's ability to fulfil them, but people do not always act according to their roles, and they are creative enough to find ways of dealing with these expectations. Therefore, an analysis of social roles does not prevent us from seeing the agency in people's actions. Secondly, as Cohen also says (1994: 27), 'the analysis of social relations calls up status and role, but not self'. This is the point I have endeavoured to make in this chapter. An understanding of the experience of infertility necessitates an understanding of social relations, because it is these relations which influence experience most. Therefore, status and role are indispensable tools of analysis. Moreover, an analysis based on the self rather than social relations in a sensitive subject such as infertility would be dangerous, in the sense that any claims made on the self of the infertile person would mean looking at who or what she is (as Cohen [1982: 10] also claims): 'infertile', 'barren', 'fruitless tree', 'dry', 'incomplete woman'. I would rather look at social interactions and show their impact on the experience of infertility by also looking at how childless women react to this impact.

Childlessness not only cuts a woman off from her social networks but also delimits the boundaries of that network. It is not only extended family members who influence the lives of childless women; neighbours are also a source of stress as well as support. This chapter discussed the ways in which neighbours with children assert the right to control childless women's lives. It remains a challenge for childless women to negotiate their female identities when having children delineates those identities.

Notes

1. In addition, according to the Dictionary of the Turkish Language Foundation, *dişi* (female) is used to refer to the sex that produces eggs or gives birth. It also implies womanly (*kadınsı*), feminine (*feminen*). It is noteworthy that being female is described by giving birth. However, this does not lead to the masculinization of infertile women.
2. Not in Dere but in more urban middle-class families, the boy's family may bring chocolate on a silver tray and flowers. These kinds of customs show a rich variety across Turkey and across social classes.
3. I did not have the chance to witness any *söz* ceremony when I was located in the two villages. I asked two of the girls whose weddings I attended about their *söz* and I got a very similar account from both of them. Firdevs from Dere also gave me a similar account of the *söz* ceremonies she witnessed.
4. This sort of abduction or elopement with the bride's consent is called 'mock bride theft' by Ayres (1974: 238) in a cross-cultural comparison and *kaçışma* in Turkish by Kudat (1974: 292) for Turkish practices.
5. Renunciation of abducting couples and the shame that falls upon an abducted bride and her parents are not only argued in Turkey. For example, see Ayres (1974) for an early cross-cultural comparison and Werner (2004, 2009) for post-Soviet Central Asia.
6. However, giving birth to a child can also be considered as an achievement when the conception is via IVF. This will be discussed later.
7. This is unlike the relationship of women with their own kin among Awlad 'Ali Bedouins in Egypt described by Abu Lughod. Awlad 'Ali women are never totally cut off from their own kin upon marriage and they feel free to return to their kin when they want to. However, a woman's identification with her kin may affect her paternal family's reputation (Abu-Lughod 1999 [1986]: 54–55).
8. I do not claim that giving a bride is not seen as a commercial transaction anywhere. I reflected on the situation in my field. Indeed, there are fathers in Turkey who give away their adolescent daughters to the man who gives the highest bride price. They make money from giving away their daughters as if they are selling their daughter as a commodity (Canoruç 2005, Kazgan 1981). According to Stirling (1965) and Kazgan (1981), the practice of bride price in Turkey compensates the bride's family for their lost labour (the daughter). In the context of North India, Sharma (1980:175) prefers to use the term bride price rather than bridewealth, as the vernacular word (*mul*) refers to price or payment. The word 'to give' (*vermek*) is usually used in Turkish rather than 'to sell' (*satmak*). However, in some places, such as Saklı in northwestern Turkey described by Ilcan (1994a: 287, 294), *satmak* is also used. For all these reasons I prefer to use 'bride price' (similar to Kazgan 1981) as a translation for the term *başlık parası* in Turkish.

9. The expenditures of the groom's family for the bride are subject to public scrutiny. For example, at Nesrin's (from Dere) henna party (bachelorette or hen night – *kına gecesi*), which took place before the wedding night, the groom's parents failed to distribute henna to the guests, contrary to custom. Many people commented on this: 'Nesrin has gone for very cheap' (*ucuza gitti*). The amount of money spent on the bride, in this respect, reflects the value given to the bride by the groom's family (this is similar to the payment of dowry by the bride's family to the groom's family, and the wedding entertainment provided by the bride's family as a means of impressing neighbours and affines in North India recounted by Sharma (1980: 143), but it is the groom's family in my field who is expected to impress others via expenditure on the bride and for the wedding). The groom's family is also expected to give jewellery as a wedding gift to the bride. There are also many other occasions on the wedding day (and before, during the preparations) when the groom is compelled to pay money to the bride's family and to others. For example, he pays money to the bride's brother when he enters the house of the bride, before he leaves the house, and while the bride's brother ties the 'virginity belt', a red ribbon which symbolizes virginity, around the bride's waist. While Nesrin's brother was expected to tie Nesrin's virginity belt, he asked for money twice. Upon the groom's complaint, he responded: 'We are *giving* you our girl, what are you talking about?'
10. '*Kan yedim, kan içtim*'. It is an idiom for suffering.
11. '*Evimize bir sıçan geldi, oramızı açan geldi, bütün gün yazıp gece okuyan geldi*'.
12. The religious marriage ceremony is not sufficient to make a couple officially married. Only civil marriage ceremonies which are conducted by the municipality are considered official. A woman who is married only via a religious ceremony cannot inherit from her late husband.
13. By the term 'neighbours', I also mean friends and acquaintances. Since it is 'neighbours' (*komşular*) who appear most in women's narratives about the people who try to control their lives by means of support or coercion, I prefer to use this word as an encompassing concept. A second popular word is *çevre*, which signifies one's immediate circle of friends and neighbours, and sometimes also relatives. Another reason for the use of 'neighbours' is to refer to the pivotal place of neighbourhood in the two villages, particularly in Village Tepe.
14. This certainly does not reflect Turkey in general. Parallel cousin marriages are typical in Turkey. See Meeker (1971) and Beller-Hann and Hann (2001) about marriage with one's father's brother's daughter (FBD) in the east Black Sea region of Turkey and Delaney (1991) about a central Anatolian village in Turkey.
15. Vaginismus refers to vaginal tightness that may prevent penetration.

16. Eating carob is a folk remedy for sexual impotency. It is considered to give one energy and 'strength'.
17. *Tohumsuz* (seedless) is another epithet for childless men. *Tohum* (the seed) is central to Delaney's (1991) ethnographic research, which took place in 1980–1982 in Central Anatolia, Turkey. The *tohum* metaphor or the despising *tohumsuz* did not come out in my own research when I inquired about the women's thoughts on procreation. I sometimes even pushed the issue so that I might provoke such epithets but this was in vain.

Chapter 4

MANHOOD IDEOLOGIES AND IVF

IVF treatment is charged with anxieties about masculinity. This chapter concerns the implications of certain manhood ideologies for the experience of childlessness and the demand for (or avoidance of) infertility treatments such as IVF.

Research in the field of assisted reproductive technologies or reproduction in general has been extensively preoccupied with women's experience of these treatments and their subjectivities (Gutmann 2009, Inhorn 2009).[1] This is not totally unexpected, because IVF 'deals directly with the female body' (Koch and Morgall 1987: 173), even if there is a male infertility factor.[2] In addition, it is usually women who face the social predicament of being childless, particularly in pronatalist settings where patriarchal ideologies dominate.[3] Furthermore, it is usually assumed that motherhood completes feminine identity for women, whereas men have other potential outlets for self-achievement such as 'employment, education, religious attainment, leisure activities, and the like' (Inhorn 2001: 93). Yet reproduction involves men as well as women, and it is imperative that men's subjectivities and manhood ideologies be considered in assessing and understanding the demand for IVF (Inhorn 2009).

The recent research focus on masculinities is evident in Inhorn's and Birenbaum-Carmeli's studies on the Middle East, especially Egypt, Israel and Lebanon.[4] An investigation into masculinities is significant especially when patriarchal ideologies dominate gender relations and inform the demand for assisted reproduction treatment. Although it is primarily women who have to endure the tribulations of infertility, women tend to shoulder the blame for infertility in the event of male infertility. This is partly due to a hegemonic manhood ideology that defines procreation as an essential proof of virility. Procreation, as I will argue, connotes something more than providing 'substance' such as sperm or ova.

Contingent Masculinities

It is important that the vernacular of gender categories be explored, since such terms reveal the articulation of power in masculine and feminine ideologies. As Cornwall and Lindisfarne (1994: 40) wrote: 'Category creation itself is an act of power'. Mainstream gender ascriptions such as man (*adam*), male (*erkek*) and masculinity (*erkeklik*), as well as woman (*kadın*), girl (*kız*), female (*dişi*), feminine (*kadınsı, dişi*), are ideologically loaded, contingent and contested categories.

The variety of terminology within the categories of masculinities is not straightforward. *Erkek* refers to a male. *Erkek* is used to differentiate physiological differences in all living things. However, *erkeklik* (maleness) in humans is also an achieved identity. One is not only born male but also has to attain maleness by proving one's manly skills. In Dere and Tepe, the most important means of attaining maleness is to prove one's sexual potency by having children. The term 'man' (*adam*) categorizes an adult male, which includes characteristics such as assuming responsibilities and behaving with appropriate manners. 'Being a man', in one sense, is also an achieved identity, but in moral terms.

The meanings attributed to gender categories in Turkey are contingent (following Gutterman 1994). They vary across regions, generations and social classes. Kandiyoti (1994: 210) gives an example of a Turkish village where there are three recognized categories for men, hinging upon age groups and concomitant expected social roles: *delikanlı* (literally, those with crazy blood) refers to young unmarried men who act out a form of masculinity that is 'untamed and undomesticated'. *Akay* refers to married adult men, and *kart akay* refers to old married men. In the two villages of Dere and Tepe, *delikanlı* is a common term whereas *akay* is not in use. The inhabitants of Village Dere who hail from the northeastern and eastern parts of Turkey use *kocaman* to refer to old men. In Tepe, the Bosnian terms for these categories vary according to age and marital status. *Muşko* indicates a male. *Monak* means an unmarried man whereas *çöyik* stands for a married man. *Star* is a name they give to old men.

In daily parlance, an idiomatic term, *erkek adam* (literally, male man) in Turkish, emphasizes the qualities regarding both being a male and a man. It is closest to the idiom of 'real man' in English. One should expect an *erkek adam* to be virile, brave, strong, honest and dependable. This idiom reinforces patriarchal gender ideologies. *Erkek adam ağlamaz* (a male man never cries) is an idiomatic example of such notions. A popular expression is *erkek adamın erkek oğlu olur* (male men have male sons). Both 'man' and 'son' are masculine nouns, but 'male' precedes both words to emphasize the significance of masculine ideals (of both being a male and having a son). In Tepe, the word equivalent to male man is *muşkarat*. Yet in that village, an expression equivalent to 'male men have male sons' does not exist; having a son – although important – is not promoted as such. The closer a man gets to these reified masculine conventions (of being an *erkek adam* and *muşkarat*), the further he positions himself away from femininity (Brittan 1989, Connell 1995: 68).

In delineating these two categories, *erkek* and *adam*, it may prove helpful to look at their negations. Referring to someone as 'not a man' (*adam değil* – in Village Tepe: *nie çöyik*) connotes an untrustworthy man who fails to achieve the moral conventions of masculinity; in other terms, a man who has not fulfilled 'secondary' expectations such as keeping promises. *Erkek değil* (not a male – in Village Tepe: *nie muşko*), is a more serious insult which implies sexual impotence and femininity. It is sometimes also employed to describe infertile men who cannot confirm their maleness by impregnating a wife.

Maleness, Manhood

For most people in the villages of Dere and Tepe, maleness is generally validated at two stages in life: through circumcision (*sünnet*) in childhood and through proving one's sexual potency in adulthood. Sexual potency may be established by the defloration of a girl on the wedding night. The custom of showing a bloodied sheet (*kanlı çarşaf*), which is practised in some parts of Turkey (Delaney 1991), is not practised in Dere and Tepe.[5] The proof of maleness is therefore established by impregnation of the wife.

In both villages, children are typically circumcised any time between the ages of five to ten. The *rite de passage* is celebrated with a party, in which the boy wears festive garments and accepts gifts along with praises such as 'Bravo, you are a male now!' (*Aferin, erkek oldun şimdi*).[6] Usually the guests are relatives, neighbours and friends of the family. I have encountered guests who come from distant parts of Turkey just to celebrate this important occasion. The parents, especially the father, are extolled as well. His friends praise the father with words such as 'so, your son is now a male'. This also connotes an implicit appraisal of the father's increasing maleness.

Circumcision makes one not only male, but also Muslim. Despite its perception as a marker of Muslim identity, circumcision is not a command in the Koran. Instead, it is *Sünnet* (Sunnah), and implies morally and practically being in line with the life of the Prophet.

Delaney (1991: 86) in the Turkish context, and Bouhdiba and Kal (2006: 27) in the Tunisian context, underline the similarity of the circumcision ritual with the wedding ceremony: both bear similar names and the structures are similar. 'In both events, circumcision and weddings, a part of the self is relinquished and sacrificed – the foreskin and the hymen – and blood is shed' (Delaney 1991: 86). In Turkish, the celebrations that take place around circumcision (*sünnet*) and marriage (*evlilik*) are called with the same word: *düğün*.[7] I concur with Bouhdiba and Kal (2006) in the symbolic valorization of the phallus in both cases. The ways in which sexual identity is attributed to a person take place are embodied, as the phallus is not only 'metaphorically present' (Bourdieu 2001: 12), but also physically: for a child an operation on his penis takes place; for an adult, his penis should be potent enough for sexual intercourse.

Hasibe is a woman I met in the North Clinic. She lives in a village close to the eastern border of Turkey and has two daughters. Her story concerns the maleness of her husband, who wants a son. In some parts of Turkey, a man who is referred to as *kirve* (or *kivre*) serves as a circumcision ritual (*sünnet*) sponsor. The decision regarding who will be the *kirve* of the circumcision ritual is usually made at the birth of a son. This custom of ritual parenthood is usually practised 'between villagers of equal age, wealth, social status, religious and ethnic origins' (Kudat 1971: 37). In this case, Hasibe's husband has been a *kirve* for the son of one of his close friends, with the expectation that his friend will be the *kirve* for his future son. Unusually, Hasibe's husband was not the social equal of his friend because he did not have a son, which is an indicator of social status where he lives. I asked Hasibe why she wanted to have IVF treatment:

> I want a boy. They will do it, won't they? I hope a boy. That's why we are here. See, the *kirve* is also ready, waiting. My husband has been a *kirve* to his son, made him male, we celebrated, gave them gold coins ... we have nothing. Tell him [the doctor], let it be a son. Can you tell the doctor? We feel ashamed, we can't say anything. You tell him, 'they want a son, don't disregard them'. We can invite the doctor to the *sünnet*. My husband will fire guns, will celebrate the male son. My husband says 'bear a son, I will fire guns everywhere, I will announce it everywhere'. I haven't been able to bear a son. I am becoming aged. What if you told the doctor about it? He would not refuse you. You will be doing a great deed. You will say 'I did something very good for a sister [*bacı*] today'.

Hasibe and her husband were anxious to have a son. He was also already well prepared for the first threshold to establish his son's maleness. They were not fully aware that sex selection was illegal in Turkey.[8]

Compulsory military service and marriage are two other contexts where socialization into masculinity takes place in the villages I studied.[9] These do not attest to competence of maleness as much as circumcision and begetting a child do; nonetheless, they contribute to the conventional ideals of masculinity. Military service is considered to be the place for boys to learn how to endure hardship and how to bear responsibilities. Military service is a site for gaining important knowledge about life, nation and modernity which makes boys into men (Sirman 1990: 31). For many, this perception of military service as the passage into adulthood and manhood also makes it a prerequisite for marriage (Sinclair-Webb 2006: 74). Marriage is the social context in which the responsibility to protect a family is attributed to men. The gendered nature of the Turkish nation (Delaney 1995) reveals the extent to which protection can be an important aspect of masculine identity. Sirman (1990: 44) notes that men and the state (masculine) are expected to protect the family (feminine) and the motherland (feminine) in Turkey. 'Man – the protector', Gilmore (1990) maintains, is encountered in much of the Mediterranean (Campbell 1964, Giovannini 1987, both cited in Gilmore 1990: 48–49). I have discussed in previous chapters the notion of man – the protector in Village Tepe.

In both of the villages, military service was a highly celebrated event. There are farewell celebrations for boys who leave home for military service. A boy's friends and male relatives go around the villages and the nearby town packed in cars, honking horns throughout the journey. They play drums and make celebratory remarks to the boy while he gets on a bus to go to the location of his military service. These celebrations are proud events for fathers, whereas they are envied by some of those who do not have sons. Mothers whose sons are in the military talk about their sons with a proud voice, despite their fear of a possible unfortunate event.

Multiple Masculinities

Turkey is a vast country where the meanings that adhere to masculinity – as with everything – show rich variety. For many people in Turkey, circumcision has ceased to be a domain of maleness. It is practised for medical reasons or as a custom. Particularly in higher socioeconomic classes in cities like Istanbul, sons are increasingly being circumcised in the first two weeks of birth, and no ceremony takes place for the circumcision. Many people do not even know what a *kirve* is, and generations grow up without seeing a single circumcision ceremony. It is the same for attributions of masculinity via deflowering or procreation. Not everyone subscribes to these values, and for some people these are bygone, 'backward' customs. There are people for whom military service is not acknowledged as a passage into manhood but as a burden that should be avoided as far as possible. Between these two extremes, there are all kinds of perceptions of the military as well as of marriage. Consequently, I would argue that there is no one uniform manhood ideology which everyone shares to the same extent in Turkey, not even in the same villages. The politics of manhood not only varies from region to region or across social classes; it can also differ within the same family.

Moreover, it is also important to historically situate these masculinities (Brittan 1989). The notions of manhood among the people with whom I did research – like any other people – are not frozen in time. The media and access to the World Wide Web also contribute to the creation and popularization of new forms of masculinities and femininities. The new kinds of masculinity discourses that propagate rapidly via the media do not necessarily perpetuate themselves. I prefer to call these 'pop masculinities' to emphasize their temporary, fashionable and swiftly consumable qualities. Since they can be powerful enough to subvert hegemonic masculine ideologies for some people at the time of their popularity, they can be considered alternative forms of hegemonic masculinities. In the long term, they also have the power to erode the hegemony of certain masculinities.

An example could be *taşfırın erkek* (literally: stone-oven male), a form of masculinity that was popularized by a sitcom, Çocuklar *Duymasın* ('The Children Should Not Hear This'). It was broadcast during 2002–2004 (on television channels *ATV* and *Star TV*, respectively), and then with a few cast changes, the sitcom started to be broadcast in 2010. *Taşfırın erkek* is a character who emphasizes the patriarchal notions of manhood: he is strong, brave, a protector, a man who identifies himself in opposition to the feminine. During the time this sitcom was shown, *taşfırın erkek* became a role model for some men who wanted to stick with patriarchal values in reaction to the move towards gender equality and acceptable forms of masculinity. The character *taşfırın erkek* became the mimetic faculty by which a sort of masculinity was mimed, only to be reproduced again by those who held the same values. In a way, mimesis of mimesis (Taussig 1993) was enacted in the evolution and persistence of an ideology of manhood.

In the same sitcom another character, referred to as *light erkek* (light male), contests these conventional masculine values. He is interested in the arts, pays attention to his appearance, and most important, he does not strive to dominate his wife. In a way, *light erkek* was a neologism of metrosexuality, which was another masculinity type promulgated by the media. Lifestyles of 'metrosexual' celebrities heavily covered in the media challenged the hegemony of the male man or *taşfırın erkek*. A metrosexual man does not adhere to the need for circumcision or impregnation of a woman to validate his masculinity. *Light erkek*'s wife in the series was called 'dominant *teyze*' (dominant aunt) by the *taşfırın erkek* to underscore the subverted gender politics performed in the matrimony.[10] In varying degrees and forms, today metrosexuality continues to erode patriarchal masculinity discourses. There are thus multiple pop masculinities that simultaneously subvert persistent masculine ideologies and create new masculinist discourses, and which are also subject to change and subversion themselves.

It is not only pop masculinities disseminated by the media that hinge upon dominant masculinities; relationships among people do not stay the same, either. Power is not a constant factor in these relationships, as discussed in the previous chapter. Mothers-in-law and daughters-in-law change, and so do their relationships; hence, the reproduction of masculine ideologies does not stay the same. Just as power is fluid and partial, so are forms of masculinity, which are a product of power contestations among men. Speaking of my research and Turkey in general, I would therefore confidently say that one could speak of 'multiple masculinities', contested, contingent, historically situated and fluid.[11]

Men's perceptions of their own masculinity can also change over a lifetime (Inhorn 2012). A man may adhere to a masculinity ideal when he is single; yet his perception of masculinity may be enhanced or transformed when he discovers he is infertile. When he has a more medicalized view of conception through familiarity with IVF, he may again alter his perception of masculinity. It is important to bear in mind that the concept of masculinity is not static; a man may exhibit multiple masculinities throughout a lifetime.

Inhorn (2012) shows that masculinity ideals and practices have been transforming in the Middle East: men are no longer totally devastated by childless marriages; love marriages (versus arranged marriages) are more common; childless men remain in their marriages with their wives whom they love; more men desire nuclear family residences. She calls these new forms of masculinities 'emergent masculinities', which are different from stereotypical Middle Eastern notions of manhood. She shows that a single concept of manhood is no longer accurate in the Middle East where there are various emergent masculinities. For the two villages Dere and Tepe, and Turkey in general, scripts of masculinities are constantly changing. To establish an exact chronology of this shift is complex, so I prefer to use the term 'multiple masculinities' rather than 'emergent masculinities'.

The concept of 'multiple masculinities' reflects a paradigm shift within the postmodernist turn in the study of masculinities. On the one hand, it may be used to refer to the multiplicity of subordinated masculinities in opposition to a dominant masculinity (for example, a hegemonic masculinity such as white heterosexual middle class, and many subordinated groups such as white working class, gay middle class, etc.). I use the term, however, to refer to many simultaneous masculinities. These multiple masculinities contest other dominant ideologies, but they are not necessarily subordinates: they are alternatives.

So far I have illustrated conventional attributions of masculinities, but I have also argued that multiple and contingent forms of masculinity exist in multiple contexts. Now I will take a different turn and emphasize the one form of masculinity I encountered most often in my research, one that has a drastic impact on the attitudes towards IVF treatment as well as on the infertility experience of both men and women.

The Conception of Homosexuality and Passivity

Hegemonic masculinity is a concept made famous by Connell (1995), who borrows the term hegemony from Gramsci's (1994) analysis of class relations. It is the name given to the type of masculinity that occupies a 'currently accepted' authority position without direct violence. It is powerful enough to dominate other masculinities and women. Connell suggests that hegemonic masculinity is always contestable, and takes place within certain gender relations. Thus there may be multiple masculinities existing within different power relations.

Connell's theory of hegemonic masculinity has garnered a great deal of criticism and he has addressed this in a recent paper (Connell and Messerschmidt 2005). A common critique is that the theory essentializes a masculinity ideal making it static and uniform (Collier 1998, Petersen 1998, 2003 and MacInnes 1998). However, this claim only applies to the essentialist applications of the concept; the conceptualization of masculinities need not be essentialist or uniform at all. Masculinities are subject to change, and may vary across classes, locations, age groups, etc. They may even vary through a man's lifetime, as specified above.

An important aspect of Connell's theory useful to my analysis is that hegemonic masculinity precludes one from getting lost in the discourse of multiple masculinities and thus overlooking masculine ideologies that persist and are reproduced in the social milieus of men, profoundly informing their lives. As Kandiyoti (2002: 277) remarks, 'dominant constructions of masculinity define the standards against which other masculinities are evaluated'. In analyzing certain hegemonic masculinities, I aim to reveal popular conceptions of infertile men.

Gutterman (1994) notes that heterosexuality is one of the two basic assumptions about men in Western culture (the other is that they are not feminist). Homophobia is described as a marker of hegemonic heterosexual masculinity in the West (Connell 1995: 78) and also in Turkey (Ertan 2008). Kandiyoti (1994: 210), speaking about the Turkish village she studied (the one given as an example of the variance in gender categories), warns against an easy elevation of gender categories to a cultural norm, as well as against positioning any variant gender enactments within these categories as deviant. However, she adds that male homosexuality always carries the risk of being subordinated as such. She notes that male homosexuality 'presents interesting puzzles for the management of masculine identities'. I would argue that the perception of male homosexuality from a hegemonic view of masculinity could offer us an understanding of the puzzle of subordination of infertile men. Procreation is still a domain of vindicating masculinity for many people, as I have articulated above. I suggest that this underpins a hegemonic form of masculinity that demands not only heterosexuality but also procreative performance. From that performance claims to power emerge.[12]

There are critical similarities in the subordinated masculinities of gay men and infertile men. Most evident is that neither group is considered 'masculine'. Connell (1995: 143), speaking of the contemporary Western world, suggests that in a patriarchal culture, gay men are understood as lacking masculinity.[13] Infertility, likewise, raises questions about a man's maleness for people who regard procreation as an essential 'ability' of being male. This ability hints at the second similarity between hegemonic perceptions of homosexuality and infertility. In order to understand it, I will first look at the ways in which homosexuality is subordinated in a few ethnographic accounts. Then turning to my own research, I will reveal the similarity between the two.

The definition of homosexuality is a contested one. It has been widely documented that not only the sex of the sexual partner but also the way in which a man engages in sexual intercourse shapes conceptions of homosexuality. Loizos (1994), who studied masculine sexualities in Greek ethnography, notes that a man is considered homosexual if he performs a passive role in intercourse. A man who performs penile penetration (*kolombaras*) – even during sex with another man – is respected as a male, whereas a man who is penetrated is severely stigmatized with an abusive word, *poushtis*. De Almeida (1996) shows that in a village in Portugal, homosexuality is perceived as a passive category that verges on femininity. Homosexuality, he states, is 'the most common fear and form of aggression'. Lancaster (2002), looking at the social construction of machismo in Nicaragua, gives a similar account of homosexuality: a homosexual – a *cochòn* – indicates a man who has a passive role in anal intercourse. A *moncochòn* or *machista* is a 'manly man' who has an active role and is never stigmatized in homosocial relations, as opposed to the 'passive' *cochòn* who is feminized. Cornwall (1994) explores 'gendered identities and gender ambiguity among *travestis* [transvestites] in Salvador, Brazil'. He argues that penile penetration defines masculinity. The *travestis*, as long as they are the 'active' ones (the ones who penetrate) during intercourse, are considered 'men'. The 'passive' are regarded as homosexual and also feminine. Cornwall (1994: 129) notes: 'It is not possession of a penis that confers "maleness". Rather, it is in the *use* of the penis to penetrate that the *travesti* crosses the boundary' (emphasis original).

In these (and various other) accounts, hegemonic heterosexual masculinity is presented in opposition to homosexuality and femininity in a very particular way. The central concern is being active, expressed here as penile penetration: in other words, who penetrates and who does not or cannot. Men who do not penetrate or who cannot, in this reckoning, are considered passive, which is seen as a feminine attribute. The central emphasis is put not on having a penis, but instead, as Cornwall suggests above, it is the performance that counts.

Substance and Performance

Here, I want to introduce the notion of impotence, and ask what happens if a man cannot 'perform', cannot use his penis. When penile penetration marks maleness, 'erectile dysfunction' – not being able to take an active part in sexual intercourse – inevitably signifies femininity and homosexuality.

In what follows, I want to draw attention to the conception of procreation in my research by juxtaposing 'substance' with 'performance'. Substance, as an analytic term, has been used in discussions of procreation as well as kinship in anthropology. Its use in kinship theory is more recent, roughly starting with Schneider (1968), who analysed blood as a substance that symbolizes American kinship.[14] In discussions of procreation, substance usually emerges as semen, seed, sperm, egg/ova/oocyte or as 'female physical substance' and 'male physical substance' that are shared with the offspring. In assisted conception, donor sperm and donor oocytes are also substances of procreation, and the transmission of substances is isolated from sexual intercourse in procreation.[15]

The term 'substance' has been met with criticism. Carsten (2001: 29–30) underlines the ambiguity in the concept because of the breadth of the meanings associated with the term, but she also argues that it is useful for the same reason. Thomas (1999: 22), on the other hand, is more reserved about this breadth of uses: by making local concepts superficially similar, there is a risk of obscuring differences. *Madde* is the Turkish equivalent of the term. The dictionary published by the Turkish Language Association gives meanings similar to the ones provided by Carsten (2001: 30) in its English usage.[16] However, the reason I borrow the term is to emphasize the contribution of this chapter's argument to existing theoretical discussions on procreation and masculinities.

The literature with regard to procreation up to now has widely singled out substance in the form of – for example – the sperm or seed, while neglecting the performance of the procreative act. This has been so at least since Malinowski, whose preoccupation with the question of who contributes which substance to the offspring had a longstanding influence on the anthropological study of procreation. Malinowski (1929) famously argued that the Trobrianders were 'ignorant' of the paternal contribution to procreation: it was only the mother who was physiologically connected to the offspring, as she was the one who fed the foetus with her blood. Although Malinowski himself wrote that a man has to 'open the way' for a pregnancy to occur, he still did not consider the male contribution in the procreation theory. This lack of attention to the male procreative contribution led to a surge of interest in the so-called 'virgin birth' debates by anthropologists.[17] Malinowski himself was ignorant of the paternal contribution due to his understanding of procreation, namely, providing substance to the offspring.[18] While he was claiming that the Trobrianders were ignorant of the father's contribution to procreation in terms of providing substance, he himself remained ignorant of the other roles played out in procreation.

Malinowski's failure to see the husband's role in procreation was pointed out by Strathern (1988: 235–240), who underlined the husband's and the wife's brother's roles in procreation. Carsten (2001: 41–44) has analysed Strathern's 'denial' of Malinowski's argument: the mother's contribution of substance to the child. I want to draw attention instead to Strathern's emphasis on the active role played by the husband and the brother in procreation. Strathern argues that the brother, who produces yams, and the mother, who produces *dala* children, cannot directly exchange with each other. The brother, thus, gives yams to the mother's husband, who 'opens the way' through sexual intercourse for the *dala* child's entry into her body at conception and who creates 'the woman's body as container'. '[I]t seems to be the husband's *activity* rather than his emissions that take effect' (Strathern 1988: 236, emphasis added). Strathern points to the active role played by the husband here for procreation. This is, she notes, different from sharing bodily emissions. Only by virtue of the sexual act can the husband contribute to procreation. Virility does not seem to be an issue here. Still, the true point of emphasis in procreation here lies in performance, rather than substance.

The emphasis on substance in procreation also pervades the procreation studies of Turkey and Egypt. For example, Delaney (1991) argues for the extreme importance of men's procreative power through providing the seed in Turkey. Inhorn (1996: 242, 2003b, 2004) explains the importance of proving virility for urban poor men in Egypt. She also notes the conflation of impotence with infertility (2003b: 238, 248). But she underscores a procreative account similar to that described by Delaney: for a man in Egypt, procreation is realized by placing worms (sperm) into a woman's womb.

My research material suggests that for people who share a certain heterosexual masculine ideology, male infertility connotes impotence. Sexual impotence, with an emphasis on the inability to penetrate, confers ambiguity on a man's maleness. Thus, infertility poses the risk of being considered feminine. So the second association drawn between a homosexual and an infertile man is the assumption of a lack of penile penetration. Here I will give an example of the perception of impotence as being homosexual and at the same time feminine. After this, I will provide examples from the narratives of women I met in the IVF clinics about the conception of male infertility as impotence.

One day, Elif and I were conversing with Hatice and her sister Esra on our balcony. They were recounting stories of women whose husbands were impotent. Upon hearing one of the stories, Elif stood up and started to strut. She was making fun of the impotent man. Walking coquettishly and laughing, she asked Hatice: 'So he was like this, a woman?' Elif was imitating gayness as well as femininity. Stereotypes of impotent and gay men plainly echoed in her mockery.[19]

Havva had been married for twenty years and had three daughters. I met her when she was having her second IVF trial in an attempt to conceive a son. Despite the fact that they had three daughters, some people still did not consider her husband male, for in their social circles, fathering a son is the ultimate confirmation of maleness. As she told me, the worst kind of insult for her and for her husband was a friend of hers belittling her husband's inability to 'make a son':

> Come on, let my husband make a child for you [*gel de sana bir çocuk yaptırsın benim beyim*]. Your husband is unable to do that. Come and

> let my husband do it for you. (38 years old, married for 20 years, second IVF cycle for a son)[20]

This was a reference to her husband's sexual performance. In one sense, conceiving a son implies better sexual performance. Although it is not very common, I have heard this kind of humiliation from others; she is not alone in hearing such contempt. 'Making a child', here, insinuates being potent enough to penetrate. Although Havva has three daughters, her husband is regarded as not performing well enough to produce a son. The emphasis here is entirely on potency.

Even if his wife has an infertility-related problem, there may be misgivings about a man's sexual potency. Since male infertility is severely stigmatized, it is known that women claim responsibility for infertility problems in order to protect their husbands. The more time passes without children, the more the sexual potency of a man, and hence his maleness, becomes contestable.

This popular perception of male infertility can disrupt childless men's subjectivities. The encounter with infertility can become extremely traumatic for men in whose social circles childlessness will cast aspersions on their masculinity. Another difficult aspect of the encounter with childlessness is the fact that it questions one's purpose in life, for it is held by many that rearing a child (or a son) is the ultimate purpose of life. Below is an example of the emotional trauma infertile men go through.

Seyra was a 27-year-old woman married for five years. When I met her at the South Clinic, she had just come out of egg retrieval for her fourth IVF trial. Seyra had never disclosed her IVF treatment to anyone since she was afraid to make her husband's infertility problem public. She was living in Istanbul, but since they were going to move to her husband's hometown in a few months, she was anxious to get pregnant. She was worried about the feelings of her husband, who had a low sperm count. Her emphasis on maleness pertains to the general depiction of infertile men suffering from sexual impotence, rather than a low sperm count:

> This raises psychological problems for my husband. It is not easy for him to know that we cannot have a child because of him. We cannot tell anyone that we are unable to have a child. People think about maleness. They think he is not male. It is totally irrelevant but people think that a childless man is not male. This bitterly distresses him ... After three years, nobody believes you do not want to have a child. So to closer people I say it is because of me [to others she says they

> do not want a child yet]. I will never tell anyone it is because of him. (27 years old, married for 5 years, male-factor infertility, fourth IVF cycle)

Homosociality (same gender relationships) is of utmost importance in determining how infertility is experienced, for the enactment of masculinity takes place in 'homosocial competition', as Inhorn (2003b, 2004, 2007b) notes regarding the Middle East. Women ascribe more importance to their husbands' subjectivities in homosocial encounters than to their own. Despite the social predicament of being an infertile woman, fertile women with infertile husbands shoulder the 'procreative blame' (Inhorn 2003b) and so have to face the social stigmatization of infertility.[21] To quote Berger et al. (1995: 7): 'Far from being just about men, the idea of masculinity engages, inflects and shapes everyone'. Shouldering the blame of infertility does not prevent a husband's maleness from being scorned.

I have frequently been told in the villages that male infertility is seldom discussed among men, as a man's insinuation about another childless man's lack of maleness provides legitimate grounds for a fight. Men may face an innuendo such as 'you must have a problem'. Taking it as a subtle insult to their maleness, they find it harder to accommodate infertility.

Nuriye (whom I interviewed at the South Clinic), married for ten years, describes the intricacies of being childless for her husband:

> Merve: Why do you think men do not tell others about their infertility problems?
> Nuriye: Male pride [*erkeklik gururu*], I reckon.[22]
> M: What does that mean?
> N: Men do not accept it. I do not know how to explain that. It may be about losing their male pride – [laughing] they are not male any more.
> ...
> M: How does your husband feel about it [being childless]?
> N: My husband says he encounters questions. His friends ask him, 'Why is there no child, there should be one'. There are a few rude colleagues who tell him 'then you have a problem'.
> M: What do they mean?
> N: Then, it means... They imply 'you are not male'. That is the meaning that comes out of it. But of course, they do not say it directly. We women can cry and laugh and can even do mad things but men always keep everything to themselves. They have bigger problems. (30 years old, married for 10 years, unexplained infertility, had artificial insemination once before)

Nuriye's words reveal the importance of 'male pride' when it comes to disclosing male infertility problems. Men are afraid of the stigma attached to male infertility and its possible ramifications in homosocial relations. Another interesting point here is Nuriye's view that 'men have bigger problems'. Contestation of her husband's male identity is seen as more important than anything a woman may experience in her social life.

While maleness is bound up with the sexual prowess of a man, a man's body structure is a sign of potency in local reckoning. It comes as no surprise, then, that well-built men are expected to have many children, including sons. I have encountered women in infertility clinics who wasted years on treatments to no avail, as their well-built (but infertile) husbands would never be considered infertile due to the association people made between physical appearance and the achievement of 'making a baby' via procreative performance.[23]

Hanife was one of these women who spent ten years having treatment despite her husband's low sperm count. She revealed this to me while she was undertaking her second round of IVF treatment. Looking at his tall and well-built body, her husband's family assumed that he did not have a problem. 'Even after we had the test results they were not convinced. They thought the test was wrong and we had to repeat it somewhere else.' His parents called her barren (*kısır*) for many years, due to the association they made between physical appearance and the achievement of 'making a baby' via performance derived from physical strength.

'Men are infertile while women have [fertility] problems' (*Erkeğin kısırı, kadının kusuru olur*). This comment, heard in the village quite a few times and twice in the infertility clinics, is quite telling. 'Infertility' or 'barrenness' (*kısırlık*), seen as a hopeless condition, is here attributed to men, not to women. Women, by this reckoning, can have reproductive problems, albeit treatable. I have been given examples of women who got pregnant with hormonal treatments as evidence. The prevalent belief is that 'problems with eggs' are difficulties of a treatable variety. Nonetheless, when it comes to men, they have two sorts of problems, both of which are incurable: they are either sexually impotent or without sperm. In either situation, the condition is considered hopeless and described as infertility. This is in stark contrast to the perception of infertility noted by Inhorn (2003b: 247): in Egypt, male infertility problems are regarded as correctable in comparison to female problems, and male infertility is rarely seen as the main reason for a couple's childlessness.

IVF and Virility

On rare occasions, TV transmissions broadcast accounts of the work of physicians who treat women with sperm that is not that of their husbands.[24] Despite their infrequency compared to the numerous informative and laudatory appearances of the treatment, these programmes are known to a great number of people. Couples usually take all possible precautions to ensure that their treatment remains secret, thus averting doubts and rumours about the identity of their IVF child's 'real father'.

As it is reported by Inhorn (2004), men in Cairo also have concerns about the perception of IVF as a treatment that makes use of sperm other than that of the husband. She notes that in Lebanon, the stigma attached to IVF has significantly decreased over the years, as IVF has become better known and more prevalent. Interestingly, this is despite the fact that unlike in Turkey and Egypt, IVF via donor sperm is possible in Lebanon. In Turkey, knowledge of IVF has also increased and IVF is stigmatized less, but it still raises questions about the father of the child for many people. This is exemplified in the following narrative from Cansel, who made it known to people that their first child was an IVF child:

> My daughter has grown up now. My husband's relatives sometimes say: 'She looks like her father. If she did not, we would be doubtful about her real father'. My husband is extremely pleased. He says: 'Thank God she looks like me. This shows what people have in their minds'. (35 years old, married for 16 years, male-factor infertility)

There are two main reasons for a childless couple to conceal IVF treatment. One is, as articulated above, the ambiguity surrounding the father of the child due to misconceptions about IVF treatment. Secondly, and probably more importantly, it will be known to others (and to the man himself) that conception did not come from the man's success in impregnating the woman. The birth of the child will be far from a vindication; his male identity will remain ambiguous. By this token, an IVF baby does not meet the expectations of men in terms of manhood ideals. In such circumstances, the father of the IVF baby is deemed infertile, impotent, not male and not even 'the father' of the baby, as epitomized above. It comes, therefore, as no surprise that the utmost care will be taken by men to avoid such a predicament.

In summary, there are palpable reasons for men's reluctance to have IVF and to refrain from disclosing the treatment to other people. Nearly all of the women I interviewed at the clinics had initiated the treatment themselves despite their husbands' disinclination towards it. In the villages as well, men were the ones who had to be persuaded to undergo IVF. Kerime was not able to convince her husband to do this when I was there. People would probably not consider her husband as 'not male' because of his tall, well-built body, but he was still cautious about creating any misunderstandings.

Cevriye's involuntarily childless daughter-in-law was complaining that her husband wanted to 'make a child' and would not agree to 'seek support'.[25] His concern about 'making a child', along with his reluctance to have IVF, hint to the fact that he does not see himself as a procreator when the child is conceived *in vitro*. If substance (his sperm) had primacy over performance (penetrating his wife) his attitude would be different, as he would still have a major role in procreation in that respect. It is competence in impregnating a wife that makes a man a procreator, as well as male.[26]

I argue that endeavours to avoid as well as to disguise IVF treatment by men are still highly prevalent, and the care given to these attempts demonstrates the significance of manhood ideologies. It underlines achieving procreation by penetration as a prerequisite for attaining and preserving maleness. I will now explore the impact of the stigma attached to male infertility on the whole family.

Total Loss

I hold that it is important to pose the question: what are the reasons for women's willingness to keep male infertility hidden, despite the adversities they may experience for years, in some cases for all their lives? The first answer to this question appeals to the patriarchal power some men enjoy. This is articulated as a 'patriarchal paradox' by Inhorn (2003b). Secondly, when a man is deemed infertile, his wife goes through social exclusion and humiliation along with him, which is even more intense in such a case.

In sum, a man's loss of male identity can become so socially intolerable that the whole family may find it difficult to accommodate such a predicament. They may choose to move to another city, where 'the problem' is not known. However, years of marriage without a child may make a man's male identity ambiguous in the new social environment as well. I call these effects of male infertility on the whole family 'total loss'. I will present a few examples of the ramifications of sexual impotence before I provide an example of a childless couple who have endured total loss due to a manhood ideology that reifies potency and procreation.

While Elif and I were having our tea on the patio with Hatice and Esra, Esra started to tell a story of a distant relative who stayed married for twelve years to a man who was sexually impotent. The woman wanted to continue her marriage to avoid having to 'go back' to her natal kin as her divorced sister had done. Going back would be a shame, a failure she did not dare face. She was also unable to disclose her marital problem. She avoided putting her husband in a difficult situation:

> The man was not male. She could not tell anyone for twelve years. When someone asked why they did not have a child, she would say it was because of her. She could never say, 'my husband is not male and he is unable to do *that*'.

Hatice interjected comments to the story while she busily embroidered a bright red headscarf:

> Her aunt, too, went through the same experience. She died without having had sexual intercourse with her husband. She could not tell a soul about it. She was saying to us that the reason for their childlessness was because of some problems she herself had. She preferred assuming the blame to having her husband disparaged. How could she say that my husband is unable to do *that*? [She laughed when she said that and continued] They could have harshly despised the man. He may not have survived. So, these two women lived as virgins.

Esra continued:

> That woman who stayed married for twelve years did not marry again. Her husband told her: 'I never touched you, I never hurt you, why are you leaving me?'

At that moment all of us burst into laughter. Esra, laughing as well, continued:

> Yes, he said that. Then the man went into decline. He went bankrupt. He lost everything. You see, a man who cannot be male, cannot be anything. If it is spoken out loud, his life is ruined. I think, not until it was disclosed, did he accept it. Otherwise, how could he live normally without being male?

'Wedding-night murder' (*gerdek gecesi cinayeti*) is an incident that occasionally takes place in Turkey when a man discovers his impotence and kills the bride who witnesses it (Lindsfarne 1994: 92). A story of a man, for instance, appeared on the news on 26 May 2008. This man was accused of shooting his bride on their wedding night, allegedly upon discovering that the bride was not a virgin. After writing on the mirror that the girl was not a virgin, he shot himself, too. The girl was saved, but he was seriously injured. The comments made about this story on various news websites are compelling. There is a prevalent presumption among readers about the man's sexual impotence, and some of them feminize the man because of that. An example: '... your penis did not work. Why did you do that to the innocent woman? Anything you do is in vain, you have nothing [no sign of potency], *pembelim* [meaning something close to: my one who wears pink]'.[27]

Here is another story, this time from Sultan, about the course of events that took place after making her and her husband's involuntary childlessness public knowledge:[28]

> My man suffered from gastric bleeding for seven years after his brothers scorned him: 'Male men have male children. People like you cannot have sons unlike us who can'. They meant that my man was a woman, hence his childlessness. Now that we are seen on television, people know that we cannot have a child. So in his workplace they told my man: 'You are *zürriyetsiz* [without offspring], you cannot have a child, we cannot accept you among us and work with you'. So he suffered from gastric bleeding again. Now he works somewhere else. There, the boss who is also his friend insulted him saying that no one other than he himself would accept him in his workplace. Now he [her husband] does not want to work anymore.

Notwithstanding the fact that her husband did not have known fertility problems, as confirmed on the television programme by the physicians who treated them, her husband's male identity was made ambiguous. When we talked on the phone a month later, she told me her husband was unemployed:

> Nobody wants to give him a job. They tell him 'you are not male'. Now I totally regret that I appeared on television. We cannot walk down the street without being insulted. Our life has been devastated since people learnt we couldn't have a child. Merve, our entire life has gone.

These stories reveal the all-encompassing consequences of sexual impotence and male infertility on the lives of men and their families. I suggest we call these totalizing outcomes 'total loss'. In so doing, I aim to underscore the impact of male infertility on all the members of the family as well as on all aspects of family life. The family members face the risk of losing their friends, jobs, the place they live, authority, prestige and their expectations of life along with their identities.

Nearly all of the women I interviewed at the clinics had initiated the treatment themselves, despite their husbands' disinclination towards it. Two of my childless friends in Village Tepe were not able to undertake IVF, as they could not convince their husbands to do so. For their husbands, the birth of an IVF child would be far from a vindication of their ordeal: their male identity would remain ambiguous until they achieved impregnation. As Strathern (1988: 65) suggests for Highlanders in Papua New Guinea, masculinity is not about having certain attributes. Sexual identity is constantly produced while performing it (Butler 1990). By the same token, infertile men who resort to IVF lack the pivotal means of performing their sexual identity. This does not imply how male identity is expressed; rather, it highlights how it is produced. Via procreation, men not only make children but also make their sexual identity. Thus when we look at men's attitudes towards IVF, following Ortner (1996), we observe actors engaging in the making or unmaking of gender.

To conclude, despite the existence of a variety of masculinities, for many, sexual potency is still a signifier of maleness, and procreation is the ultimate domain where maleness is performed. The male identities of infertile men who do not meet the standards of a hegemonic masculinity type become ambiguous. These men are excluded from the greater group of males. Belonging emerges as a social necessity without which they, along with their families, suffer total loss. Understandably, male infertility is often concealed. For those people who uphold this standard of maleness, IVF deprives men of using their procreative performance ability, and hence of an opportunity to produce their maleness.

Notes

1. This is especially true of ethnographies on Europe and North America. Becker (2000) is an exception. With regard to the Middle East, in Inhorn's (2002, 2003b, 2004, 2006a, 2006b, 2007a, 2007b, 2009, 2012) work, a careful analysis of masculine ideologies plays an important part in understanding the experience of childlessness. The papers in the

volume *Reconceiving the Second Sex* (Inhorn et al. 2009) also focus on men's experiences of infertility and IVF.

2. Men do not undergo drug treatment, and under normal conditions they do not undertake any operation. However, they provide semen through masturbation. As Inhorn (2007a: 38) remarks, this can be a profound experience, especially when it fails, and when enough living sperm cannot be provided by masturbation, they undergo surgical operations such as testicular semen extractions or aspirations. However, in my view – in contrast to Inhorn's – compared to women's experience of IVF, men's experience still remains minor in general. More importantly, this view (that women's role in IVF is more significant compared to men) is also common among men and women in this research who undergo IVF.
3. See Beller-Hann (1999) and Beller-Hann and Hann (2001) for the Lazi population in Turkey and Delaney (1991) for a central Anatolian village in Turkey, Handwerker (1995, 1998) for the Han people in Beijing, Inhorn (1994, 1996, 2001, 2003a, 2003b, 2004 among others) for Egypt and Lebanon, Gupta (2000), Neff (1994), Riessman (2000a, 2000b) and Widge (2002) for India. The previous chapter discussed this topic in the context of this research.
4. See Inhorn (2002, 2003b, 2004, 2007a, 2007b, 2009), and Inhorn and Birenbaum-Carmeli (2009a, 2009b).
5. This should not imply that virginity is not important in these villages. All men expect their brides to be virgins. This reflects the expectations of the majority of Turkish men. According to a survey (2006) conducted in seventeen cities across all regions of Turkey for a newspaper, seventy-four per cent of men in Turkey prefer that a girl remain a virgin until marriage (Armutçu 2006). Another indication of the importance attributed to virginity is 'virginity exams' (*bekaret testi*). This usually happens when the parents of a girl have doubts over the virginity of their daughter. There are sporadic appearances of incidents in the media when the girl to be examined commits suicide or encounters violence after a negative result. Parla (2001) notes that in Turkey, the discussions surrounding virginity exams take place around a modern-traditional dichotomy. She argues that the employment of virginity exams as institutionalized violence upon women's bodies and their individual rights is a product of the modernization project in Turkey, which promoted an ideal of the modern but chaste woman.
6. In using the term *rite de passage*, I indicate a ritualistic ceremony that marks the transition of a boy to a *male* child. It is a transition ritual, but somewhat different from the seminal use of the term by Van Gennep (1960 [1909]). The separation and incorporation phases are not particularly differentiated. Yet, during the ceremony, the boy might be considered to be going through a liminal (Turner 1967) stage, during which he wears an ornamented dress. Courage, which 'male men'

have, is expected from the child: he may be told 'not to cry like a girl'. A boy who goes through this in a brave manner will be applauded for being a male man (*erkek adam*). There is not much change in the boy's life after the ceremony. However, if a boy does not go through this ceremony until a certain age, he may be severely scorned about his non-male identity.

7. There may also be other similarities between the two celebrations. In the circumcision ceremonies described by Fallers and Fallers (1976: 256), a 'henna party night' (*kına gecesi*) – which usually precedes wedding ceremonies – is also organized the day before a boy is circumcised. Even though this is seen in some places in Turkey, the villagers of Dere and Tepe do not organize a henna party for circumcision.
8. Sex selection is legally possible only for medical reasons such as for avoiding the transmission of a sex-linked genetic disease.
9. In Turkey there is mandatory conscription lasting between six and fifteen months for all 'able-bodied' men over twenty years old.
10. Polat Alemdar, the leading role of a TV series *Kurtlar Vadisi* (The Valley of Wolves), could be another perfect example of a masculinity type promoted by the media. Polat Alemdar is a charismatic nationalist man who engages in murder in the interest of the state. He does not like to treat women well. This character has been extremely influential: in a survey conducted by the Association of Ankara Young Businessmen in 2008 among 1,634 young people between the ages of eighteen and thirty living in Ankara, Polat Alemdar was voted one of the top three role models (the other two were a programme host and one of the wealthiest businessmen in Turkey).
11. See the articles by Lindisfarne, Kandiyoti as well as Cornwall and Lindisfarne in *Dislocating Masculinities: Comparative Ethnographies* ed. by A. Cornwall and N. Lindisfarne (1994) for anthropological discussions on multiple masculinities.
12. This is also reflected in the vernacular of 'sexually impotent' in Turkish: *iktidarsız* (literally: without power).
13. I would rather not use 'culture' as a bounded entity and speak of its aspects, but instead would argue that in gender relations in which patriarchal ideologies operate, male homosexuality is positioned as far as possible from hegemonic heterosexual ideals.
14. In fact, substance (or the order of nature) was half of Schneider's analysis of American kinship. The other half was code (or the order of law).
15. In discussions of procreation there is usually a biogenetic substance that is transmitted to the offspring from one (monogenetic) or both (duogenetic) genders. In kinship theory, however, the substance need not be biogenetic. For example: milk – as in milk kinship – described by Clarke (2009: 40–43).

16. See the meanings of *madde* on the association's website: http://tdkterim.gov.tr/bts/?kategori=verilst&kelime=madde&ayn=tam available on 10 October 2009.
17. For example, see Leach (1967), Montague (1971) and Spiro (1968) for discussions concerning whether the Trobrianders or Australian natives had knowledge of physiological paternity or not. Delaney (1986) criticized these debates for confining paternity to physiological paternity and ignoring conceptual paternity, i.e., the relationship of cosmology to procreation. I find Delaney's critique important for underlining the constructedness of paternity and begetting. However, due to focusing only on the seed/sperm, she leaves out other possible conceptualizations of paternity such as the ones addressed in this chapter.
18. Malinowski's emphasis on substance in procreation is not unexpected. Indeed, it reflects a European approach to procreation and kinship. See Schneider for American kinship (1968) and Strathern for British kinship (1992a).
19. Being masculine, however, is not usually an insult for a woman. This is reminiscent of the esteem given to the masculine identity credentials among the Awlad'Ali Bedouins (Abu-Lughod 1999: 110–111) who tend to value the women who display traits of manly virtues such as assertiveness, strength and intelligence.
20. Havva and her husband, unlike Hasibe mentioned earlier, were not expecting to have sex-selection. They were at the clinic with the hope that God would give them a son. Their daughters had been conceived *in vivo*. They had been having trouble with conception for the last thirteen years (the youngest daughter is fourteen years old).
21. A similar tendency by women to shoulder the blame of infertility has been presented by Inhorn (1994, 1996, 2003a, 2003b) for Egypt, and by Abbasi Shavazi et al. (2008) for Iran.
22. Male pride is a common term that refers to the importance of upholding the tenets of masculinity. It appears as a reason for wanting children and for preserving male identity. It has a similar use among the urban poor in Egypt (Inhorn 1994: 61).
23. For a cross-cultural analysis of the association of 'bigness' with masculinity, see Gilmore (1990: 110). By 'bigness', Gilmore implies more than musculature. He also indicates and gives examples of 'bigness' measured in accomplishments or numbers of possessions, all associated with masculinity. According to Inhorn (2003b), male infertility conjures up a man's 'weakness' in Egypt. However, it is 'weak worms' (sperm) rather than impotence that accounts for weakness in men. For a historical overview of the association of muscularity with masculinity in the American context, see Forth (2008), who states that male physical performance, which is increasingly seen as the performance of a machine, is nowadays most harshly tested 'in the bedroom'.
24. This was also discussed in the introduction.

25. There is no direct translation of the word 'procreation' in Turkish. *Çocuk yapmak* (literally 'to make a child') would be the closest idiom to this expression. *Çocuk yapmak* can indicate procreation and impregnation as well as bearing a child in different contexts.
26. This is another major reason for men's reluctance to have IVF: their role in procreation via IVF. This will be explored in more detail in the next chapter.
27. This commentary, along with the news article, was available at the news website http://www.haberler.com/gerdek-gecesi-damat-cinneti-haberi-yorumlari/ on 7 March 2009. The title of the article is *Gerdek Gecesi Damat Cinneti* (Madness of a Groom on the Wedding Night). There are also others who have committed suicide because of sexual impotence on their wedding nights. An example of this appeared on the news on 17 August 2009. A man who married his uncle's daughter committed suicide on the wedding night due to sexual impotence. Readers' comments on the news on the website of a popular newspaper usually expressed pity for the groom. Cousin marriage was also a topic of criticism among the comments, for it was considered a sign of 'backwardness'. This was available on the website of the newspaper *Vatan*: http://w9.gazetevatan.com/Evlendigi_gun_intihar_etti/254366/7/Manset.
28. I have talked about Sultan before in Chapter 3. I met her via the producers of a morning television programme targeted at housewives. She was sponsored by that programme to have IVF treatment. She told me her story during an interview I had with her in her house and during various telephone conversations.

Chapter 5

ACHIEVEMENT AND PROCREATION

Here I will suggest a theoretical framework that reveals the ways in which women subvert dominant discourses of masculinity and femininity in their quest for achievement, and empower themselves through *in vitro* conception. In doing so, I plan to enrich the previous chapter's discussion on procreation.

In this research it was almost always women who initiated and persisted with IVF. The head of the South IVF Clinic spoke of the 'obsessive demand' of the women who came there for treatment, which occurs after one or more failed IVF cycles: 'They become determined to score a goal, ignoring any compromise in the quality of their lives'. I have also observed women (in the two IVF clinics where I did research) who persisted with the treatment despite the serious health risks involved. There were others who continued regardless of severe economic hardships. There were some who persisted despite pressure against IVF from their affines. As has been mentioned before, husbands seemed less likely to want to continue the treatment.

Women's persistence with repeated cycles of IVF has been analysed as a 'never enough' attitude (Thompson 2005: 240) and as an 'unrelenting drive' (Becker 1990: xxi). Sandelowski (1993: 41) calls women's persistence with IVF a 'magnificent obsession'. IVF has been seen as a hope technology (Franklin 1997) or as a failed technology (Klein 1989) that promises more than it delivers. Once technologies such as IVF are an option, they can produce a forced choice (Franklin 1988: 108), or prescriptive fertility (Strathern 1992a: 36–37), whereby women face pressure to try them (Franklin 1988: 107–110, 1997: 170–176) from the less than 'satisfactory' options (Stanworth 1987: 12). The calculation of the success rate of these technologies with respect to the number of cycles of IVF undergone compels their repetitive use (Sandelowski 1991, 1993: 49, Thompson 2005: 118).

Early feminist literature criticized women who persist with IVF for being subservient to patriarchal ideologies that reify and dictate motherhood (Arditti, Klein and Minden 1984, Corea 1985, Corea et al. 1987, Ratcliff 1989). The later work was cautious about the disembodiment of conception (F.V. Price 1990), and the increasing power of male practitioners over reproduction (Franklin 1995, 1997, Steinberg 1990). Women were seen as objectified by masculine technologies in the hands of men (Stolcke 1988: 117). The idea that reproduction had increasingly been appropriated by men pervaded the feminist stance in the history and philosophy of reproductive medicine (Stanworth 1987: 3).[1] In opposition to these, this chapter will further the previous chapter's argument that the disembodiment of conception in the case of IVF is more relevant for men, and instead it is women who are more empowered by conception through IVF.

Notwithstanding all of the following: hegemonic femininities and masculinities, the structure of kin relations that mandate motherhood, the emphasis on having a son, and the sanctity of motherhood in religious discourse, childless women can still resist the undesirable outcomes of childlessness with regard to power inequalities. This was evinced in the second chapter, where it was shown how childless women deployed the religious rhetoric of 'everything is God-given' to empower themselves. The third chapter scrutinized the ways women negotiated for more privacy and control in their social networks, as well as for full gender and adult identities. In the fourth chapter, women's role in managing the amount and type of information revealed about male infertility was discussed. This chapter argues that reproductive technology does not necessarily objectify women (Thompson 2005: 180). I do not intend to depict the infertile woman as a heroic sufferer (Sandelowski and de Lacey 2002: 43) who resists and transcends all gender, kin and religious conventions in order to romanticize resistance (Abu Lughod 1990). However, I want to emphasize that a childless woman, acting as a subject, may use medical technology for her empowerment. Infertile women are, as Greil (2004: 103, 111) notes in the context of infertile women in New York State, 'problem solvers, operating creatively within a system they do not control', and the women I describe below are proud of themselves for being actively involved in the treatment.

The vignettes from the narratives elicited in the two IVF clinics demonstrate the gendered attitude towards IVF. It will be apparent later that this gendered attitude to IVF stems from a gendered attitude to procreation *in vivo* and *in vitro*.[2] The vignettes below exemplify that women not only initiate treatment, but also are quite determined to continue it, regardless of their own and their husbands' social background, education level or employment status. By comparison, their husbands are likely to give up in case of a 'failure'. In none of the cases below are the problems associated with infertility solely female problems.

Narin is a 35-year-old university graduate who works as a textile designer in Istanbul. She has been married for three and a half years to a marketing manager. The couple did not want to have a child in the first couple of years. They had undertaken artificial insemination three times before I met them at their first IVF treatment. Narin is much more determined to conceive *in vitro* than her husband:

> My husband does not want a child very much. 'If we have a child, it will happen naturally, forget about it', he says. I am a bit insistent.

Mina, a 42-year-old nurse married for six years, lives close to the South Clinic where I met her. She has already gone through five cycles of IVF. Mina is so determined to conceive that she has also made use of folk remedies, although usually – as a nurse – she is opposed to them. In her previous attempts at IVF, she had one or two eggs retrieved each time, but this time sixteen eggs were retrieved after the use of folk remedies:

> My husband does not care a penny. I have not heard once from him, 'let's go to a doctor'. I have never heard it. I was always the one who instigated these treatments ... But I am not like him, I am ambitious. This will happen. I will make it done.

Nurdan, a housewife, and her husband, a worker in a shipyard, live in the outskirts of Istanbul. They had a child within the first year of their marriage. For the last twelve years, they have been trying to conceive a second child with assisted reproduction treatment:

> My husband loves children but says one is enough. He has always reacted to my insistence on a second child. He has always been opposed. He has never been beside me. I have always had these treatments through my own efforts. Even now, he is not with me.

Nesibe's husband, a vocational high school graduate, is a worker in a factory close to the South Clinic where I met them. She is a primary school graduate housewife. Her husband is not supportive of IVF:

> My husband is more fatalistic than me. It seems he has let everything take its course. In fact, he says if it is meant to be, it will be. I am not like that. I feel this desire so deep inside me. Let's say like this: I want it.

These women are determined not only for motherhood (*annelik*) but also for procreation (*çocuk yapmak*) *in vitro*, if not *in vivo*. Via *in vivo* conception, by sexual intercourse, women are not considered to be playing a major role as they do in IVF. As was also explained in the previous chapter, men have a relatively more prominent role in *in vivo* conception, but not the sole role. All the couples I met in the IVF clinics knew that for conception, sperm and ova are equally essential.

If women are held responsible for failure (infertility), it is indeed because they are also held responsible to a certain extent for success (a child). This is because they also contribute to procreation (via providing substance). Yet, the reverse is at least as true. The women I describe here are not in fact held responsible for failure because the major role for success belongs to men (performance). As was brought out in the previous chapter, I encountered the idiom, 'women have problems [related to fertility], but men are infertile'. This indicates that, in Turkey, infertility can be attributed to men.

I agree with Delaney's argument that for many, paternity means mostly begetting, while motherhood means nurturing (1986, 1991). Yet this should not mean that begetting implies only providing the seed. As was explained in the previous chapter, begetting also means being able to provide that seed, that is, being sexually potent enough. In the case of IVF, although their seed/sperm is still essential, men are no longer needed for such performance. Women, on the other hand, take the major role in IVF. They are the dedicated performers of procreation from the outset. And now that they apply the hormonal injections themselves, they have even a greater performance in the process of procreation.

Women whom I interviewed in the IVF clinics liked to express their proud feelings for having *produced a child themselves*. Suna, a woman I met and made friends with in the South Clinic, for example, never succeeded in persuading her husband to get IVF. She had to bring the sperm sample to the hospital herself, since her husband refused to come to the hospital. That was why she was alone when I met her during her egg retrieval and embryo transfer. When we talked a few weeks after she had given birth to twins, she was proud of herself for having achieved the procreation of her babies *alone* and *despite* her husband.

Most of the women emphasize the ease of the IVF treatment and disguise their fears and feelings of weakness. Only three of the women in this research complained about the injections that they had to apply themselves every day (even twice a day, for a period). None mentioned pain except for these three. I encountered a few women who highlighted the stress associated with their worries. Questions linger in their minds such as: How many eggs will be retrieved? Do we have 'high quality' and enough sperm? Will fertilization happen or not? Will the embryo stick to the uterus?[3]

Another problem pertains to the limbo they exist in during the thirteen days between the embryo transfer and the pregnancy test (Sandelowski 1993: 45). Despite the high chance of non-implantation, women may feel like they are pregnant with an embryo in their uterus. Some of them take care of themselves as if they are pregnant. As a woman who was undergoing IVF put it: 'It is as if you are pregnant for thirteen days'. That is why, when the result of the pregnancy test is negative, frustration leads to emotional breakdown.

The biggest difficulty regarding the treatment, as far as I have observed (and also noted by various research, Franklin 1997 for example), is the experience of a negative pregnancy test result, in other words, 'failing'. Some women's menstrual periods begin just before having the test. The frustration is too big to bear for many: 'I was dreaming of having a positive test result. I planned to have a pregnancy test, but before I could go to the pharmacy, my menstrual period started. Instead, I went to the pharmacy to buy a pack of menstrual pads. I cannot tell you enough how horrible it feels', narrated a friend of mine who underwent IVF.

Women who take responsibility for producing their children also take responsibility for 'failing'. They may blame themselves for working too hard after the embryo transfer, for taking it too seriously, for being too stressed, etc. Now that a 'taking it easy' discourse prevails in the success narratives, even worrying too much about the implantation can lead to self-blame. I have also met a few women who blamed their mothers-in-law. They considered themselves to have 'miscarried' their 'babies' because of their mothers-in-law who made them work excessively. When the women blamed themselves for doing too much domestic work, it was usually because they were too immaculate, giving too much importance to cleanliness, etc. The failure in being a woman due to an inability to conceive was meant to be because of an act that also indicated womanhood.

Despite these difficulties, women usually want to underline the ease of the treatment. I can see two alternative explanations for this. First, they may really find the treatment easier than they had expected. It is true that IVF is more effortless (for example the hormonal injections can be performed by women themselves) compared to when it was criticized in the feminist literature two decades ago. Yet, as seen above, the treatment still creates difficulties such as coping with stress.

A possible second explanation is that women do not want to admit any difficulty at all. This is because it is already apparent that there are hardships in the treatment, and by saying that the treatment is very easy, they stress its ease *for them*. It is a marker of their 'strength'. One of the nurses in the South Clinic also mentioned that the patients never wanted to confess that the treatment was ever difficult for them. This was also in spite of their difficulties in understanding certain parts of the treatment. For example, many semi-literate women were told how to apply the hormonal injections to their own bodies. They found it hard sometimes to understand how much of which medicine to put in the syringe and how often to inject them. Sometimes they were deeply worried about doing something incorrectly.

Sedir, whom I met at the South Clinic during an embryo transfer, has been married for twenty-two years. Even though she has a son, she has been trying to have a second child for years. Despite the fact that the treatment is highly stressful for her, she considers it 'easy':

> After the egg retrieval, we went home. We started to worry about the fertilization. What if there is no fertilization? Will they call us? What will happen now? Today, we will go home and start worrying about the implantation and pregnancy. But the treatment is easy.

Mina, the nurse mentioned above who was able to raise her number of eggs retrieved thanks to folk medicine, is proud of her robustness:

> I do not feel like I am sick. For instance, I have had the egg retrieval operation six times. I have never used painkillers. I am extremely

robust. I never use painkillers; I try to tolerate even a high level of pain. I am not like that sort of person who expects compassion from others. I am strong.

When I started my research, my initial plan was to learn the motives for motherhood in order to understand the demand for IVF. Through the course of the research I realized that it is not only motherhood that matters. The drive to initiate IVF and further, to persist with treatment, is bound up with one's attitude towards procreation and achievement. IVF has significantly influenced how women approach procreation: via IVF, the women described in this chapter have seen how much they can do to produce their children. This new role in procreation also gives women an opportunity to achieve something important in life.

So far, it has been revealed that most of the women in my research, both in the villages and in the IVF clinics, do not have the chance to achieve anything they would regard as major. Some are proud of their excellence in domestic chores or in needlework. This is truer of housewives. Yet there were also university graduates with impressive careers who complained about having achieved nothing in life.

Below are some more vignettes from the interviews conducted at the IVF clinics:

- I have fought a lot for this [*çok mücadele verdim*]. I have been distressed. My psychology has been ruined. I have had treatment for that. Yet, I never lost hope. I moved on. I said: 'There will never be a failure in this'. That there is a child on the horizon for me always lingers in my mind. I cannot live without a child. If there is no outcome from this, I will adopt a child. I have not talked about it with my husband. There is no way without a child. (39 years old, married for 13 years, male-factor infertility, shop manager)

- My husband is totally against these IVF trials for a second child. He is concerned about my health. But I am determined. I am ready to face all the risks involved. I am determined to win this battle. I want a child no matter my health. (42 years old, married for 6 years, female factor-infertility, nurse)

- There is always sorrow but I am hopeful. If this fails, I will try again, I will go as far as it takes. I am totally determined. Not until I achieve this, will I give up. I see it as a battle. I will go on hoping we win. (38 years old, married for 16 years, female-factor infertility, lawyer, third IVF trial)

– Hormones induce stress. He does not like it. 'We did not get married for children', he says, 'it was love'. I am not like him. I am ambitious. I know I will achieve it one day. I will get it done. (41 years old, married for 24 years, female-factor infertility, housewife)

– If you ask me why I want a child, for example there were people who got married the year I married, they immediately became pregnant. During the first year we did not want a child. Yet, when I learnt that we had a problem, I became extremely ambitious. My husband does not care. I did the first cycle myself and I am the one who wanted this one. I do not want to leave my child as an only child. (31 years old, married for 7 years, male-factor secondary infertility, housewife)

– There are people who struggle to conceive a child for years. For example, my uncle and his wife. I want to struggle for this as well. I know I will love the child more if it is my achievement. I will say: 'I did this. I fought for it and I made it come true'. The child will be the fruit of my battle in one sense. It will be *my* child. (23 years old, married for 3 years, female-factor infertility, was a worker in the textile industry when she was single, now a housewife)

These women are determined to produce a child regardless of the stakes, such as their health. They are determined to 'fight for it' despite their husbands' disinclination. They even seem to enjoy the fact that they are alone in this 'battle'. They are the ones who take it to the end without any help from others.[4]

The idioms of achievement, war and battle are also found in the public presentations of IVF. The stories of women who have achieved, who have 'won their battles', are deployed so that childless women are motivated to get endless treatments until they have a child, winning their battle. For example the website *cocukistiyorum.com* ('I want a child') is one of these spaces where having a child is conceptualized as a war to be won. *Savaşı kazananlar* ('The ones who have won the war') is the name of a page on this website where women who have had IVF babies write their stories. They explain how determined they had been and suggest that women should persist when they encounter obstacles or failure. The story of the founder of the website is a perfect example; she explicitly presents her story as a battle. The whole website is designed to motivate women to take IVF treatment as a war to be won and to never give up. As well as providing information about IVF treatment and IVF specialists, the website promotes a certain image of the involuntarily childless woman. This is a dedicated woman who uses all kinds of media for information and who is determined to do anything to win her battle. Achievement is a driving metaphor in this website.[5]

Achievement (*başarmak, başarı*) is a concept I was not expecting to encounter during my research. I had thought of it as a Euro-American preoccupation in the ethnographies of IVF (Franklin 1997 on the United Kingdom, Thompson 2005 on the United States). Conceiving a child as an achievement in life also appears in the narratives collected by Bonaccorso (2009: 37) at IVF centres in Milan, Italy. Achievement, for many women in my research, is a gendered concern; women are not expected to 'achieve' things in life (although they may strive for it).

Usually not until women encounter failure does achievement come to the fore. Divorce and childlessness are such failures. Both divorced and childless women such as the ones below are made to feel like failures, 'extensively discredited' in Goffman's terms (1963: 2, 3). A childless woman feels failure, for example, when a younger sister-in-law who gets pregnant humiliates her. Childless women may even feel failure when they compare themselves with an animal that can produce offspring.

Yaren lives in Adıyaman. She is a 42-year-old woman, married and childless for twenty-two years:

> Each time I see that I have a period again I start crying. I cry when I see chicks, telling myself that I am not able to be at least like a chicken ... A chicken lays out many [eggs, chicks] each time; I *cannot* do [accomplish] even one. I am not able to do even one.

Tarhan is thirty-four years old but has been a childless married woman for seventeen years. She lives in Tekirdağ, close to the northwestern border of Turkey. I interviewed her during her second IVF trial:

> You see a dog on the street, excuse me, you say, 'it has a puppy near it, you could not be as much as it'.

Eventually, feelings of incompleteness and abnormality follow. Similar to the metaphor of the fruitless tree (discussed in the first chapter), these kinds of comments reveal how childless women find themselves failing their 'nature' (physiological or biological).

The masculinity of achievement is most apparent in the narratives when women refer to having success in a 'battle' after a period of 'fighting'. Battle is a masculine metaphor for the treatment.

Fighting indicates women's efforts in that battle. It is men who serve in the military and who take part in battles, both literally and metaphorically. Women are often the ones who are expected to fulfil expectations associated with feminine roles such as being a wife, a daughter-in-law, etc. Perfection in domestic work – although it may give a sense of achievement – is praised as a marker of a 'good woman', but is never compared to winning a battle. Women, who are proud of their active role in IVF, understand that they are accomplishing a major achievement. Consequently, they feel more confident and determined in the face of challenges that may arise.

One must be willing to fight to win a battle. It is not easily won. The treatment is perceived similarly. It may take a long time – because of failed attempts – as well as taking determination and patience to endure. Women who consider the treatment as a battle welcome these hardships. Although a failed cycle is often a traumatic experience, the will to continue persists when failure is seen as a step forward in the battle. The greater and more prolonged the struggle, the greater the victory upon success. Consequently, the desire to achieve grows along with the challenges one has to cope with.

Women who endlessly pursue IVF may be reproducing patriarchal values such as the mandate of motherhood. However by appropriating attitudes and roles that usually belong to men, such as achieving victory in a battle, and being the major procreator of their child, they subvert gender conventions and even transcend them. This is more easily seen when the ethnographic artefact in focus is procreation rather than motherhood. *In vivo* procreation belongs more to men, whereas *in vitro* procreation belongs more to women.

This goes against the analysis of 'achieving conception' (Franklin 1995, 1997) in the context of England.[6] Conception is achieved in the case of IVF, she proclaims, by the involvement of many actors, including the male medical professionals and the state. In contrast, the women I am talking about do not ascribe the achievement of conception to technology or other actors but only to themselves. The achievement of conception, or to put it better, of procreation (*çocuk yapmak*), is theirs. In the procreation narratives I elicited in the IVF clinics (although it is still men who provide the sperm), 'men' are totally absent. Women engage in a 'fight' and God permits them to win the battle.

I should make a final note regarding God's involvement in procreation. Overall, it is generally accepted that it is God who gives people a child or not. Procreation happens thanks to God's will.

God wants people to seek a solution for their suffering, and this includes taking pains to undergo IVF. IVF, and the doctors who practise it, are instruments that women make use of while conforming to God's expectation from humans that they seek a cure. Relatively more devout women usually express this with the idiom: 'First God, then the doctor'. Almost all of the women, including those for whom religion is trivial, would always tell me: 'After all, it is God's will'. This rhetoric is not meant to underestimate their own role in procreation, but to acknowledge the fact that God who creates also makes procreation possible (or impossible). Women know of the contribution of both genders to conception, but as was explained in the last chapter, the work of procreation is more than a transfer of gametes; it is also performative. In these narratives, it takes place by virtue of women's efforts rewarded by God. Procreation – as the activity that leads to conceiving a child – can be conducted by women, but it occurs only with the permission of God, so creation is always by God.

Procreation, as I also argued in the last chapter, is not only comprised of a transfer of substance or gametes; it is also a performance. The question of who puts more effort into conception remains at least as important as who provides the substance. Although procreation in my research takes into account the contribution of substance by both genders, in terms of the performance role, prominence may lean towards the man or the woman depending upon context.

I find that there is too much confusion regarding God's role in procreation. Sholkamy (1999: 157) calls the Islamic view of procreation theo-genetic. In my view, God's role is not conceptualized as being confined to providing genetic substance, and hence it is not apt to infer it as theo-*genetic*. God decides who will have a child, both according to the Koran and according to the childless women I interviewed. Loizos and Heady (1999: 12) suggest that it even be called tri-genetic (male, female and God) when the act of endowing the foetus with a soul is taken into account. As I see it, giving the soul should be seen differently to giving something that carries the genetic codes of the person. Physical conception, therefore, should more aptly be called duo-genetic in the context of my research.

I do not claim in this chapter that all women share a uniform procreation theory in which they play the major role. I argued against the passive depiction of women in a masculine ART world. I found it important to note that almost all the women I met in the IVF clinics initiated the treatment themselves and pursued it despite failure. The negative side of this – reproducing the motherhood mandate which traps women in patriarchy – is often discussed in Euro-American ethnographies, as was mentioned at the beginning of this chapter.

I point to the other face of the coin. There are women who are proud to achieve procreation, which empowers them both indirectly by making them mothers and also directly through their achievement of the role of procreator. This is why they are willing to praise their determination and point to their husband's absence in the procreative process. These women have empowered themselves via procreation *in vitro*.

Notes

1. See Thompson (2005) for an overview on the feminist literature on IVF.
2. In the second chapter, there was another discussion regarding the gendered response to infertility and ART. The varying interpretations of religion and destiny by men and women were explored.
3. In fact, the questions start well before the treatment: Whether to have IVF or not, whether to have the treatment in a state or private hospital, which IVF specialist to go to, where to find the money, where to obtain information, how to make sure any treatment is appropriate in terms of religion, how to be sure how much hormonal medicine is needed, how to disguise the treatment from one's close social circles, how to get time off work for the visits to the doctor, how to decide which tests and treatments are necessary, etc. Regarding the last question, it is now popular among IVF clinics to provide certain treatment methods and additional tests to stand out from other clinics. As far as I understand these methods, some of them seem to be for marketing purposes rather than necessities for the treatment.
4. Similar metaphors for IVF treatment were also employed by the women in England (Franklin 1997: 162). Franklin notes: 'IVF pronatalism is narrated as an aggressive pursuit of an elusive goal, in which women are warriors, with battle scars attesting to their bravery on an epic quest for a child of their own. Passivity is not a virtue in the world of achieved conception'.
5. The website can be found at www.cocukistiyorum.com. It was available on 1 July 2009.
6. Franklin's research is a specific example among many other feminist studies (especially the first wave of studies) that are sensitive to increased male contribution in conception via assisted reproductive technologies. A recent example is seen in Throsby's (2004) research where achievement through IVF appears to be ascribed to medical practitioners.

CONCLUSION

I have expounded on a new perspective that examines attitudes towards the use of assisted reproduction technologies, particularly IVF. I strongly endorse the view that these attitudes are gendered. Many factors, including religion and prevalent ideologies of femininity and masculinity inform these attitudes, but these factors are also shaped by childless couples who may use them to their advantage. On the one hand, I have explored the significance of motherhood and the desire for a child. On the other hand, I have argued that the demand for IVF is more than a quest for parenthood. I have discussed patriarchal control over childless women. At the same time, I have shown the ways in which women resist this control. I argued that the gendered attitude toward procreation is a significant factor in women's persistence with IVF. Via IVF, women not only contest certain gender conventions, but also actively perform procreation. This challenges those biopolitical presumptions that represent women as desperate reproducers of patriarchal ideologies and regard medical technology as a discursive arena that appropriates feminine reproduction. What is appropriated (by IVF) is masculine procreation.

This study, looking at the experience of infertility, investigated how connections are made between gender conventions, child desire, sexuality, procreation, kinship, technology, religion, achievement and everyday experiences as well as between spaces of contestation in hegemonic discourses (of motherhood, family, religion and masculinity). It is therefore more than a study of a reproductive technology or of a biological problem. Its contribution to the anthropological studies of ART lies primarily in this multi-dimensional approach. This is especially relevant to Turkey, where Western and non-Western ways of making such connections exist together. Religion, for example, is prevalent in non-Western studies of infertility, while the concept of achievement is more common in Euro-American studies of assisted reproductive technologies. Both these elements shape the attitude of childless people towards these technologies in my research. The stigma attached to infertility appears in American (Becker 1990) ethnographies as well. However, in Turkey the scarceness of voluntary childlessness complicates stigma management and the encounter with infertility. While childlessness occurs as a challenge in both Euro-American and Turkish discourses of the family, the family takes on different meanings within the extended kinship networks discussed in this research.

This research emphasized the significance of intragender relations – especially friendship and kin networks – in power contestations and negotiations of gender and adult identity for childless women. With regards to patriarchy, this study shifted attention from the domination of women by men to the subordination of childless women by women with children in social networks.

The research findings have implications for the anthropological theory on procreation. I suggested that the significance of performance in the sexual act be underscored in investigations of procreation. The literature on masculinities is rife with depictions of homosexuality as a subordinated, feminized and stigmatized type of masculinity, but fails to acknowledge the similar subordination of infertile men. The study reveals that an investigation of manhood ideologies is essential to an understanding of the politics of infertility. This also highlights the need to think about male-imposed barriers to infertility treatments such as IVF.

The research contributes to a feminist agenda that concerns the relationship of reproductive technology and women. It emphasizes an often neglected aspect, where women act as subjects: they use religious rhetoric for empowerment, find ways to negotiate with authoritarian affines and scornful neighbours, and initiate and pursue assisted conception treatment. The book also discusses the various contexts in which these efforts are constrained, which point to the compulsion and desire behind motherhood.

Although I conducted half of my fieldwork in two villages, there is no reason to say that values attributed to children and childless people should be taken as independent from all other people in Turkey. The interviews I conducted with women from different parts of Turkey during the first half of the research show, with respect to the value attributed to children, considerable resemblance to what I observed in the villages. On the other hand, for every argument I made, it should be borne in mind that there is no one form of femininity or masculinity, and motherhood is not normative in the same way for everyone. Most importantly, although motherhood is a desire for most people, the implications of childlessness vary greatly. Class is a significant factor in delineating social pressure around childlessness in Turkey, as it is in India (Riessman 2000a, 2000b). Among the urban elite of big cities such as Istanbul, the social circles of a childless person are more likely to feel pity for the childless woman than to be contemptuous. Competition among sisters-in-law for power is seen less for various reasons: compatibility with the mother-in-law is not a vital issue, economic resources are more independent from one's family, and brothers do not necessarily live close to each other. The desire for a child is linked less to a wish to end suffering caused by others than to individual and conjugal desires. This research was more confined to underprivileged strata because those people were found more in IVF clinics (as opposed to the situation in the United States, for example, Thompson 2005) and they were more welcoming of the interviews. My knowledge of childless urban elite women derives largely from the observation of people in my own social milieu. A detailed comparison between social classes with regard to the infertility experience and demand for IVF therefore needs further research.

In order to avoid too much distraction from the core arguments, only a few of the major issues with regard to the politics of childlessness were included. In order to focus on these issues, I made limited references to other relevant and significant issues. There are also other areas of interest that need further interrogation. These are noted below.

Suggestions for Further Research

The commodification of women's bodies and gametes, gamete donation, surrogacy and the various bioethical and political implications of these practices are not addressed in this book. This is because gamete donation and surrogacy are illegal in Turkey and hence their practice very limited. Thus, a detailed discussion surrounding the implications of IVF for the perception of kinship is not included. Although such discussions practically dominate Euro-American studies on ART, there remains little published research in which comparisons to Turkey are made. An exception is a project based at the University of Humboldt, Germany, which investigated this subject between 2004 and 2012.[1] Gürtin's (2010, 2011, 2012b) work on gamete donation and reproductive tourism with regard to Turkey explores the legal, religious and moral dimensions of these practices.

Discourses produced and reproduced in the media about IVF need further scrutiny. During the period of this research, IVF was a highly popular subject in the media. IVF treatment given as a gift on many daily television programmes targeted at housewives had become a popular culture artefact. Soon after I concluded my research, specialists in nutrition and herbal medicine replaced the IVF specialists as guests on these programmes. I endorse the importance of investigating changes in biopolitical discourses. It is worth exploring the ways in which certain biomedical discourses come to the fore, along with their hegemonic reflections in the arena of reproduction. An investigation on how popular discourses on natural remedies are affecting the perception of IVF and the market for IVF is another area of interest for further research.

Stigma is an important ethnographic tool in the analysis of infertility experience in non-Western settings. A discussion in this book is not devoted to stigma, per se. On the one hand, this is because 'stigma', as a concept, does not exist in Turkish. On the other hand, the entire book reveals the stigma – as used by Goffman (1963) – attached to infertility, male infertility, IVF, sexual impotence and even failure. Nevertheless, an analysis of stigma per se might prove useful for comparison with other studies.

I confined my research to the experience of infertility rather than to the experience of IVF, which is more common in Euro-American assisted reproduction research. The body as the site of biopolitical discourse and intervention prevails in Euro-American feminist scholarly research, but I have not even touched on the subject. Instead, priority was given to the concepts that emerged from the narratives of women in the IVF clinics and in the villages. Of course, silence is also eloquent. As someone immersed in feminist and political studies about the body, I had considered it an important concern suitable for research. However, since I prioritized the concerns of my 'informants', the body as an ethnographic site lagged behind and could not find a place in this book.

Many 'faces of the state' (Navaro-Yashin 2002) are found in biopolitical discourses and practices with regards to reproduction and women, such as the legal regulations outlawing gamete donation and surrogacy, the promotion of certain femininities (roles for women) and the production and reproduction of the patriarchal family under the patriarchal state. I only make a contribution to this discussion by observing that, while the state is disguised in the discourse and practices of the 'secularist' and 'modern' IVF specialists, it is also found in the practices of the women who look for religious propriety in fertility treatment. The attitude of the couples for whom a child is essential for care in old age is one face of the state, whereas the desire to increase in number (as a family, as an ethnic minority/majority, as devout Muslims, as secularists) is another.

The political economy of infertility and IVF deserves more attention. The book does not explore in great detail the economical ramifications of infertility (and IVF) for women, in the family and in wider social networks. In that regard, the neoliberal policies regarding cuts on state funding for IVF and increased governance on the practice of assisted reproductive technologies in Turkey (e.g. the new ban on the communication between childless couples and IVF physicians regarding IVF with a third-party) need further (and urgent) contemplation. Moreover, couples who undergo treatment as loyal customers, IVF specialists, suppliers of medical technology, pharmaceutical companies and clinics have established IVF as a huge profitable market. In Turkey, IVF is now a business that brings a high return on capital, and IVF specialists earn money well above Turkish averages.[2] The proliferation of IVF clinics is therefore not only due to the high demand for IVF, and hence further research is needed on the supply side.

Concluding Remarks

I have researched the experience of infertility in order to better understand the demand for IVF. My studies indicate that the connection between infertility and demand for IVF is multifold. Since the advent of IVF, the experience of infertility has changed immensely. For example, IVF has transformed the perception of infertility from an unfortunate destiny into a curable condition.

Secondly, through regular media coverage of IVF, infertility has become a more public and 'normalized' topic. This familiarization of IVF has had various effects on the lives of childless couples. A prime example is the intrusive interest of neighbours, as discussed in the third chapter. A couple's childlessness engenders greater curiosity because of the presence of reproductive technologies. In addition to facing questions about why they are childless, couples are asked about IVF. They hear advice about going to an IVF specialist, or even about being on one of the television shows, which fund the IVF treatment of their guests. To be childless in the age of test-tube babies becomes even more difficult to explain and cope with than before this technology existed.

Thirdly, IVF has created hope for childless couples, even though it is not universally successful. Some couples lose hope after their first trial and face emotional breakdown. Others remain hopeful about IVF and continue trying for a long time, and resist building a childless life or considering adoption. Although IVF clinics and specialists are now widespread, a method for helping couples who lose hope and suffer from depression after a few unsuccessful trials of IVF has not been established. Psychological services for these couples are not common. This is perhaps because the severity of the encounter with a 'failed' cycle is not understood. For many men and women, losing hope equals losing the fundamental reason for their lives; it is socially and emotionally devastating. For women, losing the hope of having a child may equal losing hope of acceptance in their husband's family and in other social networks. It can also mean a loss of status.

Hope from IVF is also contingent upon economic factors. This hope remains inaccessible for couples who cannot afford IVF, or for women who cannot convince their husbands to go for treatment. People with the financial means can now continue to preserve their hope for a child (which may lead to greater frustration after a number of failed cycles). IVF is an expensive technology that is not available to many people due to financial constraints. State support for IVF is far from satisfactory. Some find it hard to meet the eligibility requirements for the medical report needed for state funding. For example, women must be under forty years old to apply for a medical report. Additionally, the teaching and research hospitals where these state-sponsored treatments take place are fully booked for months, and many people do not trust the quality of the service they provide. Moreover, the entire cost of the treatment and medicine is not eligible for funding, resulting in out-of-pocket expenses.

Given the condition of longing for a child that childless people endure, there will always be a demand for reproductive technologies. In the same vein, I note that it is important that the use of these technologies be contingent upon demand for them, rather than on economic inequalities. In Turkey, economic disadvantages do not stop many underprivileged people from pursuing IVF, but they have to forego their quality of life by borrowing extensive amounts of money, selling a house or even selling land, which may be the only means of income for the couple.

This book has also revealed the effect that a global technology such as IVF has had on the local realm of couples, far from the cutting-edge world where the technology was developed. Inhorn's (1996, 2003a, 2004 among others) and Clarke's (2008, 2009 among others) studies have provided examples of the ways in which IVF is received in the Muslim Middle East. As in their research, this work has shown how religion shapes people's decisions to go for IVF. It has also demonstrated the variety in the interpretation of religious discourse, and the empowering ways of using these discourses to cope with the social problems encountered in childless lives.

Another peculiarity that reveals how IVF is received in Turkey is evident in the ban on gamete and embryo donation, for the acceptance of IVF by Turkish people is also contingent upon this ban. The absence of gamete donation in Turkey is a safety valve for couples who may face suspicious inquiry. They can explain to people that third-party IVF is not possible in Turkey and hence the IVF child is 'theirs'. The practice of IVF via donor gamete or embryo would stigmatize the IVF treatment overall. Potential stigmatization comes not only from the issue of the 'legitimacy' of IVF children. Infertility, regarded as a permanent problem, can be more easily associated with people who use a donor gamete or embryo. The chances of being regarded as 'infertile' would be greater if third-party IVF were allowed in Turkey.

The encounter with IVF in Turkey also varies from the Euro-American discourses on procreation via IVF in regard to the rhetoric of the miracle. In Euro-American discussions, IVF technology is presented as a miracle to promote the superiority of science. In Turkey, the acceptance of IVF has nothing to do with the superiority of culture over nature or the miracle realized by technology. Rather, IVF babies are considered as products of the will of God, and even the technology is sometimes seen as God-given. Culture and nature thus join under the domain of God. Health specialists in Turkey are likely to avoid the rhetoric of the miracle, in a context where a miracle comes from God.

On the subject of how IVF is received in the local contexts of Turkey, there are also overlaps with the Euro-American material, such as the concept of achievement – regarding conception. In Turkey, this motive is also deliberately promoted to encourage people to go for IVF. The website cocukistiyorum.com ('I want a child'), discussed previously, is a perfect example.

Biotechnologies, when they are transferred to new locales, shape the lives of the people in those locales, who in turn shape those technologies anew. The effect of a global biotechnology once it enters the lives of people is a primary source of interest in social anthropology. Euro-American anthropological research on ART has revealed how ARTs inform the ways people conceptualize kinship and thereby themselves. In Turkey, since the practice of ART is limited to heterosexual conjugal unions, its implications may not be as far-reaching as mentioned above. Nonetheless, it still has profound effects on the lives of women and men who encounter infertility. It remains crucial, when studying ARTs, to first understand infertility, childless people and the dynamics of their social networks, and the contexts in which these technologies are received. I have aimed to accomplish that task with this book.

Notes

1. A brief description of this research is available in the introduction.
2. Income per capita in Turkey was around 7,000 USD after the global economic crisis (at the time of the research). A well-known IVF specialist earns around 400,000 USD per year.

Bibliography

Abbasi-Shavazi, M. et al. 2008. 'The "Iranian ART Revolution": Infertility, Assisted Reproductive Technology, and Third-party Donation in the Islamic Republic of Iran', *Journal of Middle East Women's Studies* 4: 1–28.

Abu-Lughod, L. 1990. 'The Romance of Resistance: Tracing Transformations of Power through Bedouin Women', *American Ethnologist* 17(1): 41–55.

———. 1999 [1986]. *Veiled Sentiments: Honour and Poetry in a Bedouin Society*. Berkeley: University of California Press.

Acar, F. 1991. 'Women in Academic Science Careers in Turkey', in F. Acar, N. Ananieva and D. Gaudart (eds), *Women in Science: Token Women or Gender Equality?* ISSC-UNESCO Publication. Oxford: Berg Publishers.

———. 1993. 'Women and University Education in Turkey', *Higher Education in Europe* 18(4): 65–77.

———. 1995. 'Women and Islam in Turkey' in Ş. Tekeli (ed.), *Women in Modern Turkish Society*. London: Zed Books.

Agarwal, B. 1997. '"Bargaining" and Gender Relations: Within and Beyond the Household', *Feminist Economics* 3(1): 1–51.

Arat, Y. 1989. *The Patriarchal Paradox: Women Politicians in Turkey*. Rutherford [NJ]: Fairleigh Dickinson University Press.

———. 2000. 'From Emancipation to Liberation: The Changing Role of Women in Turkey's Public Realm', *Journal of International Affairs* 54(1): 107–123.

Arditti, R., R.D. Klein and S. Minden (eds). 1984. *Test-tube Women: What Future for Motherhood?* London: Pandora Press.

Armutçu, E. 2006. *Türkiye'nin En Kapsamlı Cinsellik Araştırması: Türkiye Cinselliğini Konuşuyor* [The Most Extensive Research About Sexuality in Turkey: Turkey Speaks Its Sexuality]. İstanbul: Doğan Kitapçılık.

Asad, T. 1986. *The Idea of an Anthropology of Islam*. Washington, DC: Center for Contemporary Arab Studies, Georgetown University.

———. 1993. *Genealogies of Religion: Discipline and Reasons of Power in Christianity and Islam*. Baltimore: Johns Hopkins University Press.

Aswad, B.C. 1974. 'Visiting Patterns among Women of the Elite in a Small Turkish City', *Anthropological Quarterly* 47(1): 9–27.

Aydın, A. 2009. *Annee! Anne Oluyorum!* [I am Becoming a Mother!]. İstanbul: Remzi Kitabevi.

Ayres, B. 1974. 'Bride Theft and Raiding for Wives in Cross-Cultural Perspective', *Anthropological Quarterly*, Kidnapping and Elopement as Alternative Systems of Marriage (Special Issue) 47: 238–252.

Bahçeci, M. and A. Aktan. 2007. *Beni Leylek Getirmedi* [I Was Not Brought by a Stork]. İstanbul: Aura.

Bano, A. 2003. *Status of Women in Islamic Society.* New Delhi: Anmor Publications.

Basso, K.H. 1976. '"Wise Words" of the Western Apache: Metaphor and Semantic Theory', in K.H. Basso and H.A. Selby (eds), *Meaning in Anthropology*. Albuquerque: University of New Mexico Press, 93–121.

Bates, D. 1974. 'Normative and Alternative Systems of Marriage Among the Yörük of Southeastern Turkey', *Anthropological Quarterly*, Kidnapping and Elopement as Alternative Systems of Marriage (Special Issue) 47: 270–287.

Baykal, B., et al. 2008. 'Opinions of Infertile Turkish Women on Gamete Donation and Gestational Surrogacy', *Fertility and Sterility* 89: 817–822.

Becker, G. 1990. *Healing the Infertile Family: Strengthening Your Relationship in the Search for Parenthood.* Berkeley: University of California Press.

———. 1994. 'Metaphors in Disrupted Lives: Infertility and Cultural Constructions of Continuity', *Medical Anthropology Quarterly* 8(4): 383–410.

———. 1997. *Disrupted Lives: How People Create Meaning in a Chaotic World.* Berkeley: University of California Press.

———. 2000. *The Elusive Embryo: How Women and Men Approach New Reproductive Technologies*. Berkeley: University of California Press.

Behar, R. 1990. 'Rage and Redemption: Reading the Life Story of a Mexican Marketing Woman', *Feminist Studies* 16(2): 223–258.

———. 1993. *Translated Woman: Crossing the Border with Esperanza's Story.* Boston: Beacon Press.

Behar, R. and D.A. Gordon. 1995. *Women Writing Culture.* Berkeley, London: University of California Press.

Bell, S.E. 1988. 'Becoming a Political Woman: The Reconstruction and Interpretation of Experience through Stories', in A.D. Todd and S. Fisher (eds), *Gender and Discourse: The Power of Talk.* Norwood, NJ: Ablex Publishing Corporation.

Beller-Hann, I. 1999. 'Women, Work and Procreation Beliefs in Two Muslim Communities', in P. Loizos, and P. Heady (eds), *Conceiving Persons: Ethnographies of Procreation, Fertility and Growth.* London: Athlone Press, 113–137.

Beller-Hann, I. and C. Hann. 2001. *Turkish Region: State, Market and Social Identities on the East Black Sea Coast,* Santa Fe. New Mexico: School of American Research Press.

Benedict, P. 1974. 'The Kabul Günü: Structured Visiting in an Anatolian Provincial Town', *Anthropological Quarterly* 47(1): 28–47.

Berger, M., B. Wallis and S. Watson. 1995. 'Introduction', in M. Berger, B. Wallis and S. Watson (eds), *Constructing Masculinity*. New York: Routledge, 1–10.

Bertaux, D. and M. Kohli. 1984. 'Life Story Approach: A Continental View', *Annual Review of Sociology* 10: 215–237.

Birenbaum-Carmeli, D. and Y.S. Carmeli (eds). 2010. *Kin, Gene, Community: Reproductive Technologies among Jewish Israelis*. New York, Oxford: Berghahn Books.

Birenbaum-Carmeli, D. and M.C. Inhorn. 2011. *Assisting Reproduction, Testing Genes: Global Encounters with the New Biotechnologies*. New York, Oxford: Berghahn Books.

Blizzard, D. 2000. 'Situating Fetoscopy within Medical Literature and Lived Experience: An Opening for Social Analysis', in A.R. Saetnan et al. (eds), *Bodies of Technology: Women's Involvement with Reproductive Medicine*. Columbus: Ohio State University Press, 410–443.

Bonaccorso, M. 2009. *Conceiving Kinship: Assisted Conception, Procreation and Family in Southern Europe*. Oxford: Berghahn Books.

Bouhdiba, A., and A. Khal. 2006. 'Festivities of Violence: Circumcision and the Making of Men', in M. Ghoussoub, E. Sinclair-Webb (eds), *Imagined Masculinities: Male Identity and Culture in the Modern Middle East*. London: Saqi, 19–32.

Bourdieu, P. 1977. *Outline of a Theory of Practice*. Cambridge: Cambridge University Press.

———. 2001. *Masculine Domination*. Cambridge: Polity.

Brittan, A. 1989. *Masculinity and Power*. Oxford: Blackwell.

Brody, H. 1987. *Stories of Sickness*. New Haven: Yale University Press.

Bruner, J. 1986. *Actual Minds, Possible Worlds*. Cambridge, MA: Harvard University Press.

Burke, K. 1961. *The Rhetoric of Religion: Studies in Logology*. Boston: Beacon Press.

———. 1969 [1950]. *A Rhetoric of Motives*. Berkeley: University of California Press.

Busby, C. 2000. *The Performance of Gender: An Anthropology of Everyday Life in a South Indian Fishing Village*, London School of Economics Monographs on Social Anthropology, Volume 71. London: The Athlone Press.

Butler, J. 1990. *Gender Trouble: Feminism and the Subversion of Identity*. New York, London: Routledge.

Çalışlar, O. 2005. *İslamda Kadın ve Cinsellik* [Women and Sexuality in Islam]. Istanbul: Güncel Yayıncılık.

Campbell, J.K. 1964. *Honour, Family and Patronage*. Oxford: Clarendon Press.

Canoruç, M.Ş. 2005. 'Anayasa Hukuku Arasından Başlık Parası Geleneği' [Brideprice in Constitutional Law], *SBArD* 6: 233–267.

Carsten, J. 2001. 'Substantivism, Antisubstantivism and Anti-antisubstantivism' in S. Franklin and S. McKinnon (eds) *Relative Values: Reconfiguring Kinship Studies*. Durham, NC: Duke University Press, 29–53.

———. 2004. *After Kinship*. New York and Cambridge: Cambridge University Press.
Clarke, M. 2006a. 'Shiite Perspectives on Kinship and New Reproductive Technologies', *ISIM Review* 17: 26–27.
———. 2006b. 'Islam, Kinship and New Reproductive Technology', *Anthropology Today* 22: 17–20.
———. 2007a. 'The Modernity of Milk Kinship', *Social Anthropology* 15: 1–18.
———. 2007b. 'Closeness in the Age of Mechanical Reproduction: Debating Kinship and Biomedicine in Lebanon and the Middle East', *Anthropological Quarterly* 80: 379–402.
———. 2007c. 'Children of the Revolution: Ayatollah Khamene'i's "Liberal" Views on In Vitro Fertilisation', *British Journal of Middle Eastern Studies* 34: 287–303.
———. 2007d. 'Kinship, Propriety and Assisted Reproduction in the Middle East', *Anthropology of the Middle East* 2: 71–91.
———. 2008. 'New Kinship, Islam and the Liberal Tradition: Sexual Morality and New Reproductive Technology in Lebanon', *Journal of the Royal Anthropological Institute* 14: 153–169.
———. 2009. *Islam and the New Kinship: Reproductive Technology and the Shariah in Lebanon*. New York, Oxford: Berghahn Books.
Cohen, A.P. 1982. 'Belonging: The Experience of Culture' in A.P. Cohen (ed.), *Belonging: Identity and Social Organization in British Rural Cultures*. Manchester: Manchester University Press, 1–17.
———. 1994. *Self Consciousness: An Alternative Anthropology of Identity*. London and New York: Routledge.
Collier, R. 1998. *Masculinities, Crime and Criminology: Men, Heterosexuality and the Criminal(ised) Other*. London: Sage
Connell, R.W. 1995. *Masculinities*. Berkeley: University of California Press.
Connell, R.W. and J.W. Messerschmidt. 2005. 'Hegemonic Masculinity: Rethinking the Concept', *Gender and Society* 19(6): 829–859.
Connor, L. 1984. 'Comment in "The Thick and the Thin: On the Interpretive Theoretical Program of Clifford Geertz [and Comments and Reply]"', *Current Anthropology* 25: 261–280.
Corea, G. 1985. *The Mother Machine: Reproductive Technology from Artificial Insemination to Artificial Wombs*. New York: Harper and Row.
Corea, G., et al. 1987. *Man-Made Women: How New Reproductive Technologies Affect Women*. Bloomington: Indiana University Press.
Cornwall, A. 1994. 'Gendered Identities and Gender Ambiguity Among *Travestis* in Salvador, Brazil' in A. Cornwall and N. Lindisfarne (eds), *Dislocating Masculinities: Comparative Ethnographies*. London, New York: Routledge, 111–132.
Cornwall, A. and N. Lindisfarne. 1994. 'Dislocating Masculinity: Gender, Power and Anthropology', in A. Cornwall and N. Lindisfarne (eds), *Dislocating Masculinities: Comparative Ethnographies*. London, New York: Routledge, 11–47.

Crapanzano, V. 1984. 'Life Histories', *American Anthropologist* 86(4): 953–960.

Crowe, C. 1985. '"Women Want It": In Vitro Fertilization and Women's Motivations for Participation', *Women's Studies International Forum* 8: 547–552.

Cruikshank, J. 1998. *The Social Life of Stories: Narratives and Knowledge in the Yukon Territory*. Lincoln, Nebraska: University of Nebraska Press.

De Almeida, V.M. 1996. *The Hegemonic Male: Masculinity in a Portuguese Town*. Oxford: Berghahn Books.

De Kok, B.C. 2009. '"Automatically You Become a Polygamist": "Culture" and "Norms" as Resources for Normalization and Managing Accountability in Talk about Responses to Infertility', *Health (London)* 13(2): 197–217.

Delaney, C. 1986. 'The Meaning of Paternity and the Virgin Birth Debate', *Man*, New Series 21(3): 494–513.

———. 1991. *The Seed and the Soil*. Berkeley: University of California Press.

———. 1995. 'Father State, Motherhood, and the Birth of Modern Turkey', in S. Yanagisako and C. Delaney (eds), *Naturalizing Power: Essays in Feminist Cultural Analysis*. New York, London: Routledge, 177–199.

Demircioğlu, M. 2010. 'The Rhetoric of Belief and Identity in the Experience of Infertility', *Culture and Religion* 11(1): 51–67.

Duben, A. 1982. 'The Significance of Family and Kinship in Urban Turkey', in Ç. Kağıtçıbaşı (ed.), *Sex Roles, Family and Community in Turkey*. Indiana: Indiana University Turkish Studies.

Duman, Z. 1991. *Kur'an-ı Kerim ve Tıbba Göre Tüp Bebek* [Tube-baby According to the Koran and Medicine]. İstanbul: Nil Yayınları.

Ebin, V. 1994. 'Interpretations of Infertility: The Aowin People of Southwest Ghana', in C.P. MacCormack (ed.), *Ethnography of Fertility and Birth*. Illinois: Waveland Press, 131–149.

Edwards, J. 1999. 'Explicit Connections: Ethnographic Enquiry in Northwest England', in J. Edwards, S. Franklin, E. Hirsch, F. Price and M. Strathern (eds), *Technologies of Procreation: Kinship in the Age of Assisted Conception*. London: Routledge, 60–85.

———. 2000. *Born and Bred: Idioms of Kinship and New Reproductive Technologies in England*. Oxford: Oxford University Press.

———. 2004. 'Incorporating Incest: Gamete, Body and Relation in Assisted Conception', *Journal of the Royal Anthropological Institute*, N.S. 10: 755–774.

Edwards, J. and C. Salazar (eds). 2009. *European Kinship in the Age of Biotechnology*. Oxford and New York: Berghahn Books.

Edwards, J. and M. Strathern. 2000. 'Including Our Own', in J. Carsten (ed.), *Cultures of Relatedness: New Agents to the Study of Kinship*. Cambridge: Cambridge University Press, 149–166.

Ekal, B. 2006. 'How a *Kaynana* Should Behave? Discussions on the Role of Mothers-in-Law in Two *Gün* Groups', *European Journal of Turkish Studies*. Retrieved 25 May 2011 from http://ejts.revues.org/index619.html.

Ertan, C. 2008. 'Hegemonic Masculinity and Homosociality: Some Reflections on Turkey', *Ethos: Dialogues in Philosophy and Social Sciences* 1(4).

Fabian, J. 1983. *Time and the Other: How Anthropology Makes Its Object*. New York: Columbia University Press.

Fallers, L.A. and M.C. Fallers. 1976. 'Sex Roles in Edremit', in J.G. Peristiany (ed.), *Mediterranean Family Structures*. Cambridge: Cambridge University Press, 243–260.

Feldman-Savelsberg, P. 1999. *Plundered Kitchens, Empty Wombs: Threatened Reproduction and Identity in the Cameroon Grassfields*. Ann Arbor: University of Michigan Press.

———. 2002. 'Is Infertility an Unrecognized Public Health and Population Problem? The View from the Cameroon Grassfields', in M.C. Inhorn and F. Van Balen (eds), *Infertility around the Globe*. California: University of California Press, 193–214.

Fernandez, J.W. 1986. *Persuasions and Performances: The Play of Tropes in Culture*. Bloomington: Indiana University Press.

Forth, C.E. 2008. *Masculinity in the Modern West: Gender, Civilisation and the Body*. Hampshire, New York: Palgrave Macmillan.

Foucault, M. 1977. *Discipline and Punishment*. London: Tavistock.

———. 1978. *History of Sexuality, Vol. 1*. New York: Random House.

———. 1980. in C. Gordon (ed.), *Power/Knowledge: Selected Interviews and Other Writings, 1972–1977*. New York: Pantheon Books.

Frank, G. 1979. 'Finding the Common Denominator', *Ethos* 7(1): 68–94.

Franklin, S. 1988. 'Making Miracles: Scientific Progress and the Facts of Life', in S. Franklin and H. Ragone (eds), *Reproducing Reproduction: Kinship, Power and Technological Innovation*. Philadelphia: University of Pennsylvania Press, 102–117.

———. 1990. 'Deconstructing "Desperateness": The Social Construction of Infertility in Popular Representations of New Reproductive Technologies', in M. McNeil, I. Varcoe and S. Yearley (eds), *The New Reproductive Technologies*. London: Macmillan, 200–229.

———. 1995. 'Postmodern Procreation: A Cultural Account of Assisted Reproduction', in F.D. Ginsburg and R. Rapp (eds), *Conceiving the New World Order*. Berkeley: University of California Press.

———. 1997. *Embodied Progress: A Cultural Account of Assisted Conception*. London: Routledge.

Franklin, S. and M. McNeil (eds). 1998. *Reproducing Reproduction*. Philadelphia: University of Pennsylvania Press.

Freidson, E. 1970. *Profession of Medicine: A Study of Applied Knowledge*. New York: Harper and Row Publishers.

Friese, C., G. Becker and R.D. Nachtigall. 2006. 'Rethinking the Biological Clock: Eleventh Hour Moms, Miracle Moms and Meanings of Age-related Infertility', *Social Science and Medicine* 63: 1550–1560.

Gacinski, L., E. Yuånksel and H. Kentenich. 2002. 'The Unfulfilled Desire for a Child of Oriental Couples – Infertility Counselling and Treatment of Turkish Immigrants in Germany', in B. Strauß (ed.), *Involuntary Childlessness: Psychological Assessment, Counselling and Psychotherapy*. Bern: Hogrefe and Huber Publishers.

Geertz, C. 1993. 'Religion as a Cultural System', in *The Interpretation of Cultures: Selected Essays*. London: Fontana Press, 87–125.

Gilmore, D.D. 1987. *Honour and Shame and the Unity of the Mediterranean*. Washington, DC: American Anthropological Association.

———. 1990. *Manhood in the Making: Cultural Concepts of Masculinity*. New Haven and London: Yale University Press.

Giovannini, M. 1987. 'Female Chastity Codes in the Circum-Mediterranean: Comparative Perspectives' in D.D. Gilmore (ed.), *Honour and Shame and the Unity of the Mediterranean*. Washington, DC: American Anthropological Association, Special Pub. No. 22, 61–74.

Goffman, E. 1963. *Stigma: Notes on the Management of Spoiled Identity*. Englewood Cliffs, NJ: Prentice Hall.

Goldberg, S. 1975. 'Response to Leacock and Livingston: Discussion and Debate', *American Anthropologist* 77(1): 69–74.

Goodstein, E.S. 2005. *Experience Without Qualities: Boredom and Modernity*. Stanford, California: Stanford University Press.

Gramsci, A. 1994. *Letters from Prison*, trans. R. Rosenthal, ed. F. Rosengarten. New York: Columbia University Press.

Greil, A.L. 1991. *Not Yet Pregnant: Infertile Couples in Contemporary America*. New Brunswick: Rutgers University Press.

———. 1997. 'Infertility and Psychological Distress: A Critical Review of the Literature', *Social Science and Medicine* 45: 1679–1704.

———. 2004. 'Infertile Bodies: Medicalization, Metaphor, and Agency', in M.C. Inhorn and F. Van Balen (eds), *Infertility around the Globe*. California: University of California Press, 101–118.

Gupta, J.A. 2000. *New Reproductive Technologies, Women's Health and Autonomy: Freedom or Dependency?* Indo-Dutch Series on Development Alternatives 25. New Delhi: Sage.

Gutmann, M.C. 2009. 'The Missing Gamete? Ten Common Mistakes or Lies about Men's Sexual Identity', in M.C. Inhorn et al. (eds), *Reconceiving the Second Sex: Men, Masculinity, and Reproduction*. New York, Oxford: Berghahn Books, 21–44.

Gutterman, D. 1994. 'Postmodernism and the Interrogation of Masculinity', in H. Brod and M. Kauffman (eds), *Theorizing Masculinities*. Thousand Oaks, CA: Sage, 219–238.

Gülekli, B. 2006. *99 Sayfada Tüp Bebek* [Tube-baby in 99 Pages] *Söyleşi* [Interview]: D. Ünsal. İstanbul: Türkiye İş Bankası Yayınları.

Gümüşoğlu, F. 1996. *Ders Kitaplarında Cinsiyetçilik* [Gender Bias in Textbooks]. İstanbul: Kaynak.

Gürtin Z.B. 2009. '"Anything to Become a Mother": Migrant Turkish Women's Experiences of Involuntary Childlessness and Assisted Reproductive Technologies in London', in L. Culley, N. Hudson and F. van

Rooij (eds), *Marginalised Reproduction: Ethnicity Infertility and Reproductive Technologies*. London: Earthscan.

———. 2010. 'Problems with Legislating against Reproductive "Tourism"', *Commentary for BioNews*: 550.

———. 2011. 'Banning Reproductive Travel: Turkey's ART Legislation and Third-party Assisted Reproductive Reproduction', *Reproductive BioMedicine Online* 23: 555–564.

———. 2012a. 'Assisted Reproduction in Secular Turkey: Regulation, Rhetoric, and the Role of Religion', in M. Inhorn and S. Tremayne (eds), *Islam and Assisted Reproductive Technologies*. New York: Berghahn Books.

———. 2012b. 'Localizing IVF in Turkey: Practitioners as Interface Agents Between the Local and the Global', in M. Knect, M. Klotz and S. Beck (eds), *Reproductive Technologies as Global Form*. Berlin: Campus Verlag.

Haelyon, H. 2006. '"Longing for a Child": Perceptions of Motherhood among Israeli-Jewish Women Undergoing In Vitro Fertilization Treatments', *A Journal of Jewish Women's Studies and Gender Issues* 12: 177–202.

Hamdy, S. 2009. 'Islam, Fatalism, and Medical Intervention: Lessons from Egypt on the Cultivation of Forbearance (*sabr*) and Reliance on God (*tawakkul*)', *Anthropological Quarterly* 82: 173–196.

Handwerker, L. 1995. 'The Hen that Can't Lay an Egg', in J. Terry and J. Urla (eds) *Deviant Bodies: Critical Perspectives on Difference in Science and Popular Culture*. Bloomington and Indianapolis: Indiana University Press.

———. 1998. 'The Consequences of Modernity for Childless Women in China: Medicalization and Resistance', in M. Lock and P.A. Kaufert (eds), *Pragmatic Women and Body Politics*. Cambridge: Cambridge University Press, 178–205.

———. 2002. 'The Politics of Making Modern Babies in China: Reproductive Technologies and the "New" Eugenics', in M.C. Inhorn and F. Van Balen (eds), *Infertility around the Globe*. California: University of California Press, 193–214.

Hart, K. 2007. 'Love by Arrangement: The Ambiguity of "Spousal Choice" in a Turkish Village', *Journal of Royal Anthropological Institute* (N.S.) 13: 345–362.

Hartman, H. 1979. 'Capitalism, Patriarchy and Job Segregation by Sex' in Z. Eisentein (ed.), *Capitalist Patriarchy and the Case for Socialist Feminism*. New York: Monthly Review Press.

Hastrup, K. 1989 n.d. 'Writing Ethnography: State of the Art', ASA Annual Conference, Anthropology and Autobiography, York.

———. 1990. 'The Ethnographic Present: A Reinvention', *Cultural Anthropology* 5(1): 45–61.

Hatemi, H. 1999. *İlahi Hikmette Kadın*. İstanbul: Birleşik Yayıncılık.

Herzfeld, M. 1980. 'Honour and Shame: Problems in the Comparative Analysis of Moral Systems', *Man*, New Series 15(12): 339–351.

———. 1984. 'The Horns of the Mediterranean Dilemma', *American Ethnologist* 11: 439–454.

———. 1987. *Anthropology through the Looking Glass: Critical Ethnography in the Margins of Europe*. Cambridge: Cambridge University Press.
Hobart, M. 1999. 'As They Like It: Overinterpretation and Hyporeality in Bali', in R. Dilley (ed.), *The Problem of Context*. New York: Berghahn Books, 105–144.
Holmes, H., B. Hoskins and M. Gross (eds). 1981. *The Custom-Made Child: Women-Centred Perspectives*. Clifton, NJ: Humana Press.
Ilcan, S. 1994a. 'Marriage Regulation and the Rhetoric of Alliance in Northwestern Turkey', *Ethnology* 33(4): 273–296.
———. 1994b. 'Peasant Struggles and Social Change: Migration, Households and Gender in a Rural Turkish Society', *International Migration Review* 28(3): 554–579.
———. 1996. 'Fragmentary Encounters in a Moral World: Household Power Relations and Gender Politics', *Ethnology* 35(1): 33–49.
Inhorn, M.C. 1994. *Quest for Conception: Gender, Infertility and Egyptian Medical Traditions*. Philadelphia: University of Pennsylvania Press.
———. 1996. *Infertility and Patriarchy: The Cultural Politics of Gender and Family Life in Egypt*. Philadelphia: University of Pennsylvania Press.
———. 2001. 'Money, Marriage and Morality: Constraints on IVF Treatment Seeking among Infertile Egyptian Couples', in C.M. Obermeyer (ed.), *Cultural Perspectives on Health*. Oxford: Oxford University Press, 83–100.
———. 2002. 'Sexuality, Masculinity, and Infertility in Egypt: Potent Troubles in the Marital and Medical Encounters', in L. Ouzgane (ed.), Special Issue on African Masculinities, *Journal of Men's Studies* 10(3): 343–359.
———. 2003a. *Local Babies, Global Science: Gender, Religion, and In Vitro Fertilization Treatment in Egypt*. New York: Routledge.
———. 2003b. '"The Worms Are Weak": Male Infertility and Patriarchal Paradoxes in Egypt', *Men and Masculinities* 5(3): 236–256.
———. 2004. 'Middle Eastern Masculinities in the Age of New Reproductive Technologies: Male Infertility and Stigma in Egypt and Lebanon', *Medical Anthropological Quarterly* 18(2): 162–182.
———. 2006a. 'He Won't Be My Son: Middle Eastern Muslim Men's Discourses of Adoption and Gamete Donation', *Medical Anthropology Quarterly* 20(1): 94–120.
———. 2006b. 'Making Muslim Babies: IVF and Gamete Donation in Sunni versus Shi'a Islam', *Culture, Medicine and Psychiatry* 30: 427–450.
———. 2007a. 'Masturbation, Semen Collection and Men's IVF Experiences: Anxieties in the Muslim World', *Body & Society* 13(3): 37–53.
———. 2007b. 'Masculinity, Reproduction, and Male Infertility Surgery in the Middle East', *Journal of Middle East Women's Studies* 3(3): 1–20.
———. (ed.). 2007c. *Reproductive Disruptions: Gender, Technology, and Biopolitics in the New Millennium*. New York, Oxford: Berghahn Books.
———. 2009. 'Male Genital Cutting: Masculinity, Reproduction, and Male Infertility Surgeries in Egypt and Lebanon', in M.C. Inhorn et al. (eds),

Reconceiving the Second Sex: Men, Masculinity and Reproduction. New York, Oxford: Berghahn Books, 253–278.

———. 2012. *The New Arab Men: Emergent Masculinities, Technologies and Islam in the Middle East*. New York, Oxford: Berghahn Books.

Inhorn, M.C. and D. Birenbaum-Carmeli. 2009a. 'Masculinity and Marginality: Palestinian Men's Struggles with Infertility in Israel and Lebanon', *Journal of Middle East Women's Studies* 5(2): 23–52.

———. 2009b. 'Male Infertility, Chronicity, and the Plight of Palestinian Men in Israel and Lebanon' in L. Manderson and C. Smith-Morris (eds), *Chronic Conditions, Fluid States: Globalization and the Anthropology of Illness*. New Brunswick: Rutgers University Press.

Inhorn, M.C. et al. (eds). 2009. *Reconceiving the Second Sex: Men, Masculinity and Reproduction*. New York, Oxford: Berghahn Books.

Inhorn, M.C. and F. Van Balen (eds). 2001. *Infertility around the Globe: New Thinking on Childlessness, Gender and Reproductive Technologies*. Berkeley: University of California Press.

Inhorn, M.C. and S. Tremayne. 2012. *Islam and Assisted Reproductive Technologies: Sunni and Shia Perspectives*. New York and Oxford: Berghahn Books.

Işıkoğlu, M. et al. (eds). 2006. 'Public Opinion Regarding Oocyte Donation in Turkey: First Data From a Secular Population Among the Islamic World', *Human Reproduction* 21(1): 318–323.

Isvan, N.A. 1991. 'Productive and Reproductive Decisions in Turkey: The Role of Domestic Bargaining', *Journal of Marriage and the Family* 53(4): 1057–1070.

Jenkins, G.L. 2002. 'Childlessness, Adoption, and *Milagros de Dios* in Costa Rica', in M.C. Inhorn and F. Van Balen (eds), *Infertility around the Globe*. California: University of California Press, 171–189.

Joseph, S. 1993. 'Connectivity and Patriarchy among Urban Working-Class Arab Families in Lebanon', *Ethos* 21(4): 452–484.

Kahn, S.M. 2000. *Reproducing Jews: A Cultural Account of Assisted Reproduction in Israel*. Durham and London: Duke University Press.

Kağıtçıbaşı, Ç. 1982a. 'Introduction', in Ç. Kağıtçıbaşı (ed.), *Sex Roles, Family and Community in Turkey*. Indiana: Indiana University Turkish Studies.

———. 1982b. 'Value of Children and Fertility in Turkey', in Ç. Kağıtçıbaşı (ed.), *Sex Roles, Family and Community in Turkey*, Indiana: Indiana University Turkish Studies.

———. 1982c. 'Old-age Security Value of Children: Cross-Cultural Socioeconomic Evidence', *Journal of Cross-Cultural Psychology* 13: 29–42.

Kandiyoti, D. 1988. 'Bargaining with Patriarchy', *Gender and Society* 2(3): 274–290.

———. 1989. 'Women and Household Production: The Impact of Rural Transformation in Turkey', in K.P. Glavanis (ed.), *The Rural Middle East*. London: Zed Press.

———. 1991a. 'Introduction', in D. Kandiyoti (ed.), *Women, Islam and the State*. London: Macmillan.

———. 1991b. 'End of Empire: Islam, Nationalism and Women in Turkey' in D. Kandiyoti (ed.), *Women, Islam and the State*. London: Macmillan.
———. 1991c. 'Women, Islam and the State', *Middle East Report* 173: 9–14.
———. 1991d. 'Islam and Patriarchy: A Comparative Perspective' in N. Keddie and B. Baron (eds), *Shifting Boundaries: Women and Gender in Middle Eastern History*. New Haven: Yale University Press.
———. 1992. 'Women, Islam and the State: A Comparative Approach', in J.R. Cole (ed.), *Comparing Muslim Societies*. Ann Arbor: University of Michigan.
———. 1994. 'Paradoxes of Masculinity: Some Thoughts on Segregated Societies', in A. Cornwall and N. Lindisfarne (eds), *Dislocating Masculinities*. London, New York: Routledge, 197–213.
———. 2002. 'Pink Card Blues: Trouble and Strife at the Crossroads of Gender', in D. Kandiyoti and A. Saktanber (eds), *Fragments of Culture*. New Brunswick: Rutgers University Press, 277–291.
Kazgan, G. 1981. 'Labour Participation, Occupational Distribution, Educational Attainment and the Socio-Economic Status of Women in the Turkish Economy', in N. Abadan-Unat (ed.), *Women in Turkish Society*. Leiden: E.J. Brill.
Keesing, R.M. 1985. 'Conventional Metaphors and Anthropological Metaphysics: The Problematic of Cultural Translation', *Journal of Anthropological Research* 41: 201–217.
Kefeli, M. 2008. *Gökyüzünden Pencereme Sarkarken Aşk*. İstanbul: Goa.
Kim, M. 1996. 'Changing Relationships between Daughters-in-Law and Mothers-in-Law in Urban South Korea', *Anthropological Quarterly* 69(4): 179–192.
Klein, R.D. (ed.). 1989. *Infertility: Women Speak Out Their Experiences of Reproductive Medicine*. London: Pandora Press.
Knecht, M., M. Klotz and S. Beck (eds). 2012. *Reproductive Technologies as Global Form: Ethnographies of Knowledge, Practices and Transnational Encounters*. Chicago: University of Chicago Press.
Koch, L. and J. Morgall. 1987. 'Towards a Feminist Assessment of Reproductive Technology', *Acta Sociologica* 30(2): 173–191.
Konrad, M. 2005. *Nameless Relations*. New York, Oxford: Berghahn Books.
Kudat (Sertel), A. 1971. 'Ritual Kinship in Eastern Turkey', *Anthropological Quarterly* 44(1): 37–50.
———. 1974. 'Institutional Rigidity and Individual Initiative in Marriages of Turkish Peasants', *Anthropological Quarterly*, Kidnapping and Elopement as Alternative Systems of Marriage (special issue) 47(3): 288–303.
Kuhn, R. 1976. *The Demon of Noontide: Ennui in Western Literature*. New Jersey: Princeton University Press.
Lakoff, G. and M. Johnson. 1980. *Metaphors We Live By*. Chicago: The University of Chicago Press.
Lancaster, R. 2002. 'Subject Honour, Object Shame', in R. Adams and D. Savran (eds), *The Masculinities Reader*. Massachusetts: Blackwell, 41–68.

Lasker, J.N. and S. Borg. 1987. *In Search of Parenthood: Coping with Infertility and High-tech Conception*. Boston: Beacon Press.

Layne, L. 1999. *Transformative Motherhood: On Giving and Getting in a Consumer Culture*. New York and London: New York University Press.

Leach, E. 1957. 'The Epistemological Background to Malinowski's Empiricism', in R. Firth (ed.), *Man and Culture*, London: Routledge and Kegan Paul.

———. 1967. 'Virgin Birth', in *Genesis as Myth and Other Essays*. London: Cape, 85–112.

Leacock, E.B. 1963. 'Introduction', in E.B. Leacock (ed.), *Lewis Henry Morgan, Ancient Society*. New York: Meridian Books, i–xx.

Lee, R. and R. Daly 1987. 'Man's Domination and Woman's Oppression: The Question of Origins', in M. Kaufman (ed.), *Essays by Man on Pleasure, Power and Change*. Toronto, New York: Oxford University Press, 30–44.

Leonard, L. 2002. 'Problematizing Infertility: Scientific Accounts and the Chadian Women's Narratives', in M.C. Inhorn and F. Van Balen (eds), *Infertility around the Globe*. California: University of California Press, 193–214.

Limberis, V. 2000. 'Religion as the Cipher for Identity: The Cases of Emperor Julian, Libanius and Gregory Naziansus', *The Harvard Theological Review* 93(4): 373–400.

Lindisfarne, N. 1994. 'Variant Masculinities, Variant Virginities: Rethinking "Honour and Shame"', in A. Cornwall and N. Lindisfarne (eds), *Dislocating Masculinities: Comparative Ethnographies*. London, New York: Routledge, 82–96.

Llobera, J.R. 1986. 'Fieldwork in Southwestern Europe: Anthropological Panacea or Epistemological Straitjacket?', *Critique of Anthropology* 6(2): 25–33.

Loizos, P. 1994. 'A Broken Mirror: Masculine Sexuality in Greek Ethnography', in A. Cornwall and N. Lindisfarne (eds), *Dislocating Masculinities: Comparative Ethnographies*. London, New York: Routledge, 66–81.

Loizos, P. and P. Heady. 1999. 'Introduction', in P. Loizos and P. Heady (eds), *Conceiving Persons: Ethnographies of Procreation, Fertility and Growth*. London: Athlone Press, 1–17.

MacInnes, J. 1998. *The End of Masculinity: The Confusion of Sexual Genesis and Sexual Difference in Modern Society*. Buckingham: Open University Press.

Mahmood, S. 2005. *Politics of Piety: The Islamic Revival and the Feminist Subject*. Princeton and Oxford. Princeton University Press.

Malinowski, B. 1929. *The Sexual Life of Savages in North-Western Melanesia*. London: Geo. Routledge and Sons.

Marranci, G. 2008. *The Anthropology of Islam*. London and New York: Berg Publishers.

Mauss, M. 1990 [1950]. *The Gift* (translation by W.D. Halls). New York: W.W. Norton.

McQuillan, et al. 2003. 'Frustrated Fertility: Infertility and Psychological Distress Among Women', *Journal of Marriage and Family* 65: 1007–1018.

Meeker, M. 1970. *The Black Sea Turks: A Study of Honour, Descent and Marriage*, PhD dissertation. Chicago: University of Chicago.

———. 1971. 'The Black Sea Turks: Some Aspects of Their Ethnic and Cultural Background', *International Journal of Middle East Studies* 2(4): 318–345.

Mernissi, F. 2003 [1975]. *Beyond the Veil: Male-Female Dynamics in Muslim Society*. London: Saqi.

Mishler, E.G. 1986. *Research Interviewing: Context and Narrative*. Cambridge, MA: Harvard University Press.

Mitchell, L.M. and E. Georges. 2000. 'Cross-Cultural Cyborgs: Greek and Canadian Women's Discourses on Foetal Ultrasound', in A.R. Saetnan, N. Oudshoorn and M.S.M. Kirejczyk (eds), *Bodies of Technology: Women's Involvement with Reproductive Medicine*. Columbus: Ohio State University Press, 384–409.

Montague, S. 1971. 'Trobriand Kinship and the Virgin Birth Controversy', *Man* 6: 353–368.

Morgan, L.M. 2000. 'Magic and a Little Bit of Science: Technoscience, Ethnoscience, and the Social Construction of the Foetus', in A.R. Saetnan, N. Oudshoorn and M.S.M. Kirejczyk (eds), *Bodies of Technology: Women's Involvement with Reproductive Medicine*. Columbus: Ohio State University Press, 355–367.

Musharbash, Y. 2007. 'Boredom, Time and Modernity: An Example from Aboriginal Australia', *American Anthropologist* 109(2): 307–317.

Navaro-Yashin, Y. 2002. *Faces of the State: Secularism and Public Life in Turkey*. New Jersey: Princeton University Press.

Neff, D.L. 1994. 'The Social Construction of Infertility: The Case of the Matrilineal Nayars in South India', *Social Science and Medicine* 39(4): 475–485.

Neyzi, L. 1994. 'Reviewed Work(s): The Seed and the Soil: Gender and Cosmology in Turkish Village Society by Carol Delaney', *American Ethnologist* 21(1): 212–213.

Obadia, L. 2007. 'On Geertz and the Definition of Religion: The Politics of Rituals and the Economy of Symbols in the Asian Context', *Islam Re-Observed: Clifford Geertz at Morocco Conference, Dec. 06–09*. Los Angeles: UCLA Centre for Near Eastern Studies.

Ortner, S. 1984. 'Theory in Anthropology since the Sixties', *Comparative Studies in Society and History* 26(1): 126–166.

———. 1996. *Making Gender: The Politics and Erotics of Culture*. Boston: Beacon.

Özkan, M. and B. Baysan. 2006. 'Emotional Distress of Infertile Women in Turkey', *Clinical and Experimental Obstetrics & Gynaecology* 33(1): 44–46.

Parla, A. 2001. 'The "Honour" of the State: Virginity Examinations in Turkey', *Feminist Studies* 27(1): 65–88.

Pashigian, M.J. 2002. 'Conceiving the Happy Family: Infertility and Marital Politics in Northern Vietnam', in M.C. Inhorn and F. Van Balen (eds), *Infertility around the Globe*. California: University of California Press, 134–151.

Patterson, M. 2005. 'Introduction: Reclaiming Paradigms Lost', *Australian Journal of Anthropology* 16: 1–17.

Peristiany, J.G. (ed.). 1965. *Honour and Shame: The Values of Mediterranean Society*. London: Weidenfeld and Nicholson.

Petersen, A. 1998. *Unmasking the Masculine: 'Men' and 'Identity' in a Sceptical Age*. London: Sage.

———. 2003. 'Research on Men and Masculinities: Some Implications of Recent Theory for Future Work', *Men and Masculinities* 6(1): 54–69.

Pfeffer, N. 1987. 'Artificial Insemination, In Vitro Fertilisation and the Stigma of Infertility', in M. Stanworth (ed.), *Reproductive Technologies: Gender, Motherhood and Medicine*. Cambridge: Polity, 81–97.

Pina Cabral, J. de. 1989. 'The Mediterranean as a Category of Regional Comparison: A Critical View', *Current Anthropology* 30: 399–406.

Pitt-Rivers, J. 1965. 'Honour and Social Status', in J.G. Peristiany (ed.), *Honour and Shame: The Values of Mediterranean Society*, pp. 19–77. London: Weidenfeld and Nicholson.

———. 1977. *The Fate of Shechem or the Politics of Sex: Essays in the Anthropology of the Mediterranean*. Cambridge: Cambridge University Press.

Price, F.V. 1990. 'The Management of Uncertainty in Obstetric Practice: Ultrasonography, In Vitro Fertilisation and Embryo Transfer', in M. McNeil, I. Varcoe and S. Yearley (eds), *The New Reproductive Technologies*. Houndmills: Macmillan, 123–153.

Price, N. 1998. 'Institutional Determinants of High Fertility in Gwembe Tonga Society', *Social Sciences in Health* 4(1): 25–41.

Ragone, H. 1994. *Surrogate Motherhood: Conception in the Heart*. Boulder, Oxford: Westview Press.

Rapp, R. 1999. *Testing the Women, Testing the Foetus*. New York, London: Routledge.

Rassam, A. 1980. 'Women and Domestic Power in Morocco', *International Journal of Middle East Studies* 12(2): 171–179.

Rasuly-Paleczek, G. 1996. 'Some Determinants on the Study of Household Composition and Intra-Family Relations in Rural and Urban Turkey', in G. Rasuly-Paleczek (ed.), *Turkish Families in Transition*. Frankfurt am Main: Peter Lang.

Ratcliff, K.S. (ed.). 1989. *Healing Technology: Feminist Perspectives*. Ann Arbor: University of Michigan Press.

Riessman, C.K. 1987. 'When Gender is Not Enough: Women Interviewing Women', *Gender and Society* 1: 172–207.

———. 1988. 'Worlds of Difference: Contrasting Experience in Marriage and Narrative Style', in A.D. Todd and S. Fisher (eds), *Gender and Discourse: The Power of Talk*. Norwood, NJ: Ablex Publishing Corporation.

———. 1993. *Narrative Analysis*, Qualitative Research Methods Series, No. 30. Newbury Park: Sage.

———. 2000a. 'Even If We Don't Have Children, We Can Live', in C. Mattingly and L.C. Garro (eds), *Narrative and Cultural Construction of Illness and Healing*. Berkeley: University of California Press.

———. 2000b. 'Stigma and Everyday Resistance Practices: Childless Women in South India', *Gender and Society* 14(1): 111–135.

Robinson, J.A. 1981. 'Personal Narratives Reconsidered', *Journal of American Folklore*, 58–85.

Rosaldo, R. 1993. 'Notes Toward a Critique of Patriarchy from a Male Position', *Anthropological Quarterly* 66(2): 81–86.

Russell, C. 2010. 'Four Million Test-Tube Babies and Counting', *Atlantic*, retrieved 7 October 2010 from http://www.theatlantic.com/technology/archive/2010/10/four-million-test-tube-babies-and-counting/64198/.

Saktanber, A. 1993. 'Türkiye'de Medya'da Kadın: Serbest, Müsait Kadın veya İyi Eş, Fedekar Anne' [Women in Turkish Media], in Ş. Tekeli (ed.), *1980'ler Türkiye'sinde Kadın Bakış Açısından Kadınlar* [Women from Women's Point of View in 1980s Turkey]. İstanbul: İletişim Yayınları, 211–232.

Sandelowski, M. 1991. 'Compelled to Try: The Never-Enough Quality of Conceptive Technology', *Medical Anthropological Quarterly*, New Series 5: 29–47.

———. 1993. *With Child in Mind: Studies of Personal Encounter with Infertility*. Philadelphia: University of Pennsylvania Press.

Sandelowski, M. and S. de Lacey. 2002. 'The Uses of a "Disease": Infertility as Rhetorical Vehicle', in M. Inhorn and F. Van Balen (eds), *Infertility Around the Globe: New Thinking on Childlessness, Gender and Reproductive Technologies*. Berkeley: University of California Press, 33–51.

Sanjek, R. 1991. 'The Ethnographic Present', *Man*, N.S. 26(4): 609–628.

Schneider, D. 1968. *American Kinship: A Cultural Account*. Englewood Cliffs, NJ: Prentice-Hall.

———. 1972. 'What is Kinship All About?' in P. Reining (ed.), *Kinship Studies in the Morgan Centennial Year*. Washington DC: Anthropological Society of Washington, 32–63.

———. 1984. *A Critique of the Study of Kinship*. Ann Arbor: University of Michigan Press.

Selvi, D. 2007. *Delil ve Örnekleriyle Kadın ve Aile İlmihali* [Religious Guidebook about Women and Children with Proofs and Examples]. İstanbul: Pozitif.

Shankman, P. 1984. 'Comment in "The Thick and the Thin: On the Interpretive Theoretical Program of Clifford Geertz" [and Comments and Reply]', *Current Anthropology* 25: 261–280.

Sharma, U. 1980. *Women, Work, and Property in North-West India*. London: Tavistock.

Sholkamy, H.M. 1999. 'Procreation in Islam: A Reading from Egypt of People and Texts', in P. Loizos and P. Heady (eds), *Conceiving Persons: Ethnographies of Procreation, Fertility and Growth*. London: Athlone Press, 139–159.

Simic, A. 1983. 'Machismo and Cryptomatriarchy: Power, Affect, and Authority in the Contemporary Yugoslav Family', *Ethos* 11(1–2): 66–86.

Sinclair-Webb, E. 2006. '"Our Bülent is Now a Commando": Military Service and Manhood in Turkey', in M. Ghoussoub and E. Sinclair-Webb (eds), *Imagined Masculinities: Male Identity and Culture in the Modern Middle East*. London: Saqi Essentials.

Sirman, N. 1988. *Peasants and Family Farms: The Position of Households in Cotton Production in a Village of Western Turkey*, PhD dissertation. London: University of London.

———. 1989. 'Feminism in Turkey: A Short History', *New Perspectives on Turkey* 3(1): 1–34.

———. 1990. 'State, Village and Gender in Western Turkey', in A. Finkel and N. Sirman (eds), *Turkish State, Turkish Society*. London and New York: Routledge, 21–51.

———. 1993. 'Reviewed Work(s): The Seed and the Soil: Gender and Cosmology in Turkish Village Society by Carol Delaney', *American Anthropologist* N.S. 95(2): 508–509.

Soffer, Y. and D. Birenbaum-Carmeli. 2010. 'Sperm Donation in Israel: Secrecy and Anonymity', *Andrologie* 20(1): 11–19.

Spacks, P.A.M. 1995. *Boredom: The Literary History of a State of Mind*. Chicago: University of Chicago Press.

Spiro, M. 1968. 'Virgin Birth, Parthenogenesis, and Physiological Paternity', *Man* 3: 242–261.

Ssorin-Chaikov, N. 2006. 'On Heterochrony: Birthday Gifts to Stalin, 1949', *Journal of the Royal Anthropological Institute* (N.S.) 12: 355–375.

Stanworth, M. 1987. 'Reproductive Technologies and the Deconstruction of Motherhood', in M. Stanworth (ed.), *Reproductive Technologies: Gender, Motherhood and Medicine*. Minneapolis: University of Minnesota Press, 12–35.

Steinberg, D.L. 1990. 'The Depersonalization of Women through the Administration of In Vitro Fertilisation', in M. McNeil, I. Varcoe and S. Yearley (eds), *The New Reproductive Technologies*. Houndmills: Macmillan, 74–122.

Stirling, P. 1965. *Turkish Village*. New York: John Wiley and Sons.

Stolcke, V. 1988 'New Reproductive Technologies: The Old Quest for Fatherhood', *Reproductive and Genetic Engineering* 1(1): 5–19.

Strathern, M. 1988. *The Gender of the Gift: Problems with Women and Problems with Society in Melanesia*. Berkeley: University of California Press.

———. 1990 [1987]. 'Introduction', in M. Strathern (ed.), *Dealing with Inequality: Analysing Gender Relations in Melanesia and Beyond*. Cambridge: Cambridge University Press, 1–32.

———. 1991a. *Partial Connections*. Maryland: Rowman and Littlefield.

———. 1991b. 'Disparities of Embodiment: Gender Models in the Context of the New Reproductive Technologies', *Cambridge Anthropology* 15(2): 25–43.

———. 1992a. *Reproducing the Future: Anthropology, Kinship and New Reproductive Technologies*. New York: Routledge.

———. 1992b. 'The Meaning of Assisted Kinship', in M. Stacey (ed.), *Changing Human Reproduction: Social Science Perspectives*. London: Sage, 119–147.

———. 1992c. *After Nature: English Kinship in the Late Twentieth Century*. Cambridge: Cambridge University Press.

———. 1994. 'New Certainties for Old? The Case of an Enabling Technology', paper presented at the University of Lancaster, Centre for the Study of Cultural Values.

———. 1995. 'Displacing Knowledge: Technology and the Consequences for Kinship', in F.D. Ginsburg and R. Rapp (eds), *Conceiving the New World Order, The Global Politics of Reproduction*. California: University of California Press.

———. 1996. 'Cutting the Network', *Journal of the Royal Anthropological Institute* 2(3): 517–535.

———. 2005. *Kinship, Law and the Unexpected: Relatives Are Always a Surprise*. Cambridge: Cambridge University Press.

Svendson, F.L. 2005. *A Philosophy of Boredom*. London: Reaktion Books.

Taussig, M. 1993. *Mimesis and Alterity*. New York, London: Routledge.

Tekeli, Ş. 1992. '"İstanbul'da Kadın" Üzerine' [About 'Women in Istanbul']. İstanbul 3.

Terry, J. 1989. 'The Body Invaded: Medical Surveillance of Women as Reproducers', *Socialist Review* 19: 13–43.

Thiessen, I. 1999. 'The Essence of Being: Procreation and Sexuality in Mid-Century Macedonia', in P. Loizos and P. Heady (eds), *Conceiving Persons: Ethnographies of Procreation, Fertility and Growth*. London and New Brunswick: Athlone Press, 177–199.

Thomas, P. 1999. 'No Substance, No Kinship? Procreation, Performativity and Temanambondro Parent-Child Relations', in P. Loizos and P. Heady (eds), *Conceiving Persons: Ethnographies of Procreation, Fertility and Growth*. London: Athlone Press.

Thompson [Cussins], C. 1998. 'Producing Reproduction: Techniques of Normalization and Naturalization in Infertility Clinics', in S. Franklin and H. Ragone (eds), *Reproducing Reproduction: Kinship, Power and Technological Innovation*. Philadelphia: University of Pennsylvania Press, 66–101.

———. 2005. *Making Parents: The Ontological Choreography of Reproductive Technologies*. Cambridge, MA: MIT Press.

Throsby, K. 2004. *When IVF Fails: Feminism, Infertility and the Negotiation of Normality*. Basingstoke: Palgrave Macmillan.

Tremayne, S. 2006. 'Not All Muslims are Luddites', *Anthropology Today* 22(3): 1–2.

Turner, V. 1967. 'Betwixt and Between: The Liminal Period in Rites de Passage', in *The Forest of Symbols*. Ithaca, NY: Cornell University Press.

Van Gennep, A. 1960 [1909]. *The Rites of Passage*. Chicago: University of Chicago Press.

Van Rooij, F.B., F. Van Balen and J.M.A. Hermanns. 2006. 'Migrants and the Meaning of Parenthood: Involuntary Childless Turkish Migrants in The Netherlands', *Human Reproduction* 21: 1832–1838.

———. 2007. 'Emotional Distress and Infertility: Turkish Migrant Couples Compared to Dutch Couples and Couples in Western Turkey', *Journal of Psychosomatic Obstetrics and Gynaecology* 28: 87–95.

Varisco, D.M. 2005. *Islam Obscured: The Rhetoric of Anthropological Representation*. New York: Palgrave Macmillan.

Vera-Sanso, P. 1990. 'Dominant Daughters-in-Law and Submissive Mothers-in-Law? Cooperation and Conflict in South India', *Journal of the Royal Anthropological Institute* 5(4): 577–593.

Vergin, N. 1985. 'Social Change and the Family in Turkey', *Current Anthropology* 26(5): 571–574.

Wagner, R. 1986. *Symbols that Stand for Themselves*. Chicago: The University of Chicago Press.

Walby, S. 1989. 'Theorising Patriarchy', *Sociology* 23(2): 213–234.

Waters, M. 1989. 'Patriarchy and Viriarchy: An Exploration and Reconstruction of Concepts of Masculine Domination', *Sociology* 23(2): 193–211.

Weber, M. 1978. *Economy and Society*. Berkeley: University of California.

Werner, C. 2004. 'Women, Marriage, and the Nation-state: The Rise of Nonconsensual Bride Kidnapping in Post-Soviet Kazakhstan' in P.J. Luong (ed.), *Reconceptualizing Central Asia: States and Societies in Formation*. Ithaca, NY: Cornell University Press, 59–89.

———. 2009. 'Bride Abduction in Post-Soviet Central Asia: Making a Shift towards Patriarchy Through Local Discourses of Shame and Tradition', *Journal of the Royal Anthropological Institute* (N.S.) 15: 314–331.

White, J. 1994. *Money Makes Us Relatives*. Austin: University of Texas Press.

WHO. 2004. DHS Reports 9.

———. 2009. 'The Revised Glossary for Assisted Reproduction Technology (ART) Terminology', *Fertility and Sterility* 92(5).

Widge, A. 2002. 'Sociocultural Attitudes towards Infertility and Assisted Reproduction in India', in E. Vayena, P.J. Rowe and P.D. Griffin (eds), *Current Practices and Controversies in Assisted Reproduction*. Geneva: WHO.

Wikan, U. 2000. 'With Life in One's Lap: The Story of an Eye/I (or Two)', in C. Mattingly and L.C. Garro (eds), *Narrative and the Cultural Construction of Illness and Healing*. Berkeley and Los Angeles: University of California Press, 212–236.

Yaraman, A. 1999. *Türkiye'de Kadınların Siyasal Temsili* [Political Representation of Women in Turkey]. İstanbul: Bağlam.

Online Resources

Articles 7–18 of the By-law for Centres for Assisted Reproduction, Official Gazette, 19.11.1996, retrieved from http://www.mevzuat.adalet.gov.tr/html/20272.html.

Article 17 of the By-law for Centres for Assisted Reproduction, Official Gazette, 19 November 1996, retrieved from http://www.mevzuat.adalet.gov.tr/html/20272.html.

Çelebi, E. 2011. 'SGK Kesenin Ağzını Açtı, Türkiye Tüp Bebekte Dünya Yedincisi Oldu' [SGK (Social Security Association) Started Spending More, Turkey Became the Seventh in IVF in Global Ranking], *Hürriyet*, 13 February 2011. Retrieved 15 March 2011 from http://www.hurriyet.com.tr/yazarlar/17008882_p.asp. http://cocukistiyorum.com [I want a child.com].

'Çocuklar için Koruyucu Ortam: Kurumlar, Politika ve Çocuk Bakımı' [Protective Environment for Children: Institutions, Politics and Childcare], retrieved 1 May 2013 from http://www.unicef.org.tr/tr/content/detail/70/institutions-policy-and-childcare-2.html.

'Emir Komutayla Sevişilmez' [It is not Possible to Make Love on Command], interview with Dr. Mustafa Bahçeci by Elif Ergu, *Pazar Vatan*, 28 December 2008. Retrieved 28 December 2008 from http://pazarvatan.gazetevatan.com/haberdetay.asp?hkat=1&hid=13347&yaz=GpercentFCncel.

'Evlendiği Gün İntihar Etti' [He Committed Suicide on the Day of his Marriage], *Vatan*, 17 August 2009. Retrieved 20 October 2009 from http://w9.gazetevatan.com/Evlendigi_gun_intihar_etti/254366/7/Manset.

'*Gerdek Gecesi Damat Cinneti*' [Madness of a Groom on his Wedding Night], 26 May 2008. Retrieved 7 May 2009 from http://www.haberler.com/gerdek-gecesi-damat-cinneti-haberi-yorumlari/.

HFFA (Human Fertilization and Embryology Authority) Code of Practice 2009 (the section on multiple births), retrieved 3 March 2009 from http://www.hfea.gov.uk/401.html#mandatoryDirections.

KSGM (*Türkiye Cumhuriyeti Kadın Statüsü Genel Müdürlüğü*, Turkish Republic Prime Ministry Directorate General on the Status of Women), retrieved 13 December 2007 from http://www.ksgm.gov.tr/index.php.

'*Meral Okyay'la Söyleşi*' [An Interview with Meral Okyay], retrieved 23 March 2007 from http://www.vatanim.com.tr/root.vatan?exec=cikolata_detay&hkat=1&hid=10477.

Nisa Sura, Presidency of Religious Affairs, retrieved 1 October 2008 from http://www.diyanet.gov.tr/Kuran/meal.asp?page_id=83.

'*Spermci Profesöre Hapis Cezası*' [Sperm-Swapping Professor Gets Prison Sentence], *Milliyet*, 24 November 2006. Retrieved 10 February 2006 from http://www.milliyet.com.tr/2006/11/24/son/sontur26.asp.

Şura Sura, Center for Muslim-Jewish Engagement, USC (Shakir), retrieved 12 March 2009 from http://www.usc.edu/schools/college/crcc/engagement/resources/texts/muslim/quran/042.qmt.html.

Turkish Language Association Dictionary Online, definition for *sıkıntı* available at http://tdk.org.tr/TR/SozBul.aspx?F6E10F8892433CFFAAF6AA849816B2EF05A79F75456518CA.
'*Yine O Sözü Söyledi*' [He Said the Same Thing Again], *Vatan*, 5 November 2008. Retrieved 5 November 2008 from http://haber.gazetevatan.com/haberdetay.asp?detay=Erdogan_israrli_207273_9&Newsid=207273.
Legislation with regards to IVF, Prime Ministry of Turkish Republic, 29 September 2008. Retrieved 2 October 2009 from http://rega.basbakanlik.gov.tr/eskiler/2008/09/20080929M1-1.htm.
Vakıa Sura, University of Michigan, retrieved 1 July 2009 from http://quod.lib.umich.edu/cgi/k/koran/koran-idx?type=DIV0&byte=845981.

Index

www.ingramcontent.com/pod-product-compliance
Ingram Content Group UK Ltd.
Pitfield, Milton Keynes, MK11 3LW, UK
UKHW021838100926
8556IPUK00004B/422

9 781782 386346